MENTAL HEALTH–SUBSTANCE USE

Introduction to Mental Health–Substance Use

Edited by

DAVID B COOPER

Sigma Theta Tau International: The Honor Society of Nursing Award
Outstanding Contribution to Nursing Award
Editor-in-Chief, Mental Health and Substance Use: dual diagnosis
Author/Writer/Editor

Radcliffe Publishing
Oxford • New York

Radcliffe Publishing Ltd
18 Marcham Road
Abingdon
Oxon OX14 1AA
United Kingdom

www.radcliffepublishing.com
Electronic catalogue and worldwide online ordering facility.

British Library Cataloguing in Publication Data

A catalogue record for this book is available from the British Library.

ISBN-13: 978 184619 339 2

The paper used for the text pages of this book
is FSC certified. FSC (The Forest Stewardship
Council) is an international network to promote
responsible management of the world's forests.

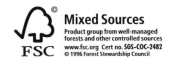

Mixed Sources
Product group from well-managed
forests and other controlled sources
www.fsc.org Cert no. SGS-COC-2482
© 1996 Forest Stewardship Council

Typeset by Pindar NZ, Auckland, New Zealand
Printed and bound by TJI Digital, Padstow, Cornwall, UK

Contents

Preface

Approximately six years ago Phil Cooper, then an MSc student, was searching for information on mental health–substance use. At that time, there was one journal and few published papers. This led to the launch of the journal, *Mental Health and Substance Use: dual diagnosis*, published by Taylor and Francis International. To launch the journal, and debate the concerns and dilemmas of psychological, physical, social, legal and spiritual professionals, Phil organised a conference for Suffolk Mental Health NHS Trust and Taylor and Francis. The response was excellent. An occurring theme was that more information, knowledge and skills were needed – driven by education and training.

Discussion with international professionals indicated a need for this type of educational information and guidance, in this format, and a proposal was submitted for one book. The single book progressed to become a series of six! The concept is that each book will follow on from the other to build a sound basis – as far as is possible – of the important approaches to mental health–substance use. The aim is to provide a 'how to' series that will be interactive with case studies, reflective study and exercises – you, as individuals and professionals, will decide if this has been achieved.

So, why do we need to know about mental health–substance use? International concerns related to interventions, and the treatment of people experiencing mental health–substance use problems, are frequently reported. These include:

➤ 'the most challenging clinical problem that we face'.[1]
➤ 'substance misuse is usual rather than exceptional amongst people with severe mental health problems'.[2]
➤ 'Mental health and substance use problems affect every local community throughout America'.[3]
➤ 'The existence of psychiatric comorbidities in young people who abuse alcohol is common, especially for conditions such as depression, anxiety, bipolar disorder, conduct disorder and attention-deficit/hyperactivity disorder'.[4]
➤ 'Mental and neurological disorders such as depression, schizophrenia, epilepsy and substance abuse . . . cause immense suffering for those affected, amplify people's vulnerability and can lead individuals into a life of poverty'.[5]

There is a need to appreciate that mental health–substance use is now a concern for us all. This series of books will bring together what is known (to some), and what is not (to some). If undertaken correctly, and you, the reader will be the judge – and those individuals you come into contact with daily will be the final judges – each book will build on the other and be of interest for the new, and the not so new, professional.

The desire to provide services that facilitate best practice for mental health–substance use is not new. The political impetus for this approach to succeed now exists. We, the professionals, need to seize on this momentum. We need to bring about the much-needed change for the individual who experiences our interventions and treatment, be that political will because of a perceived financial benefit or, as we would hope, the need to provide therapeutic interventions for the individual. Whatever the motive, now is the time to grasp the initiative.

Before we (the professionals) can practice, research, educate, manage, develop or purchase services, we must commence with knowledge. From that, we begin to understand. We commence using our new-found skills. We progress to developing the ability to examine practice, to put concepts together, to make valid judgements. We achieve this level of expertise though education, training and experience. Sometimes, we can use our own life experiences to enhance our skills. But knowledge must come first, though is often relegated to last! Professionals (from health, social, spiritual and legal backgrounds) – be they students, practitioners, researchers, educators, managers, service developers or purchasers – are all 'professionals' (in the eye of the individual we meet professionally), though each has differing depths of knowledge, skills and expertise.

What we need to remember is that the individual (those we offer care to), family and carers bring their own knowledge, skills and life experiences – some developed from dealing with ill health. The individual experiences the illness, lives with it, manages it – daily. Therefore, to bring the two together, individual and professional, to make interventions and treatment outcome effective, to meet whatever the individual feels is acceptable to his or her needs, requires mutual understanding and respect. The professionals' skills and expertise *'are founded on nothing less than their complete and perfect acceptance of one, by another'.*[6]

David B Cooper
August 2010

REFERENCES

1 Appleby L. *The National Service Framework for Mental Health: five years on.* London: Department of Health; 2004. Available at: www.dh.gov.uk/prod_consum_dh/groups/dh_digitalassets/@dh/@en/documents/digitalasset/dh_4099122.pdf (accessed 25 February 2010).
2 Department of Health. *Mental Health Policy Implementation Guide: dual diagnosis good practice guide.* 2002. Available at: www.substancemisuserct.co.uk/staff/documents/dh_4060435.pdf (accessed 25 February 2010).
3 Substance Abuse and Mental Health Service Administration. *Results from the 2008 National Survey on Drug Use and Health.* 2008. Available at: www.oas.samhsa.gov/nsduh/2k8nsduh/2k8Results.cfm (accessed 25 February 2010).
4 Australian Government. *Australian Guidelines to Reduce Health Risks from Drinking Alcohol.* 2009. Available at: www.nhmrc.gov.au/publications/synopses/ds10syn.htm (accessed 25 February 2010).
5 World Health Organization. *Mental Health Improvements for Nations Development: the WHO MIND Project.* 2008. Available at: www.who.int/mental_health/policy/en (accessed 25 February 2010).
6 Thompson F. *Lark Rise to Candleford: a trilogy.* London: Penguin Modern Classics; 2009.

About the Mental Health–Substance Use series

The six books in this series are:
1 *Introduction to Mental Health–Substance Use*
2 *Developing Services in Mental Health–Substance Use*
3 *Responding in Mental Health–Substance Use*
4 *Intervention in Mental Health–Substance Use*
5 *Care in Mental Health–Substance Use*
6 *Practice in Mental Health–Substance Use*

The series is not merely for mental health professionals but also the substance use professionals. It is not a question of 'them' (the substance use professional) teaching 'them' (the mental health professional). It is about sharing knowledge, skills and expertise. We are equal. We learn from each fellow professional, for the benefit of those whose lives we touch. The rationale is that to maintain clinical excellence, we need to be aware of the developments and practices within mental health *and* substance use. Then, we make informed choices; we take best practice, and apply this to our professional role.[1]

Generically, the series *Mental Health–Substance Use* concentrates on concerns, dilemmas and concepts specifically interrelated, as a collation of problems that directly or indirectly influence the life and well-being of the individual, family and carers. Such concerns relate not only to the individual but also to the future direction of practice, education, research, service development, interventions and treatment. While presenting a balanced view of what is best practice today, the books aim to challenge concepts and stimulate debate, exploring all aspects of the development in treatment, intervention and care responses, and the adoption of research-led best practice. To achieve this, they draw from a variety of perspectives, facilitating consideration of how professionals meet the challenges now and in the future. To accomplish this we have assembled leading, international professionals to provide insight into current thinking and developments, from a variety of perspectives, related to the many varying and diverse needs of the individual, family and carers experiencing mental health–substance use.

Reference

1 Cooper DB. Editorial: decisions. *Ment Health Subst Use*. 2010; **3**: 1–3.

About the editor

David B Cooper
Sigma Theta Tau International: The Honor Society of Nursing Award
Outstanding Contribution to Nursing Award
Editor-in-Chief: *Mental Health and Substance Use: dual diagnosis*
Author/Writer/Editor
The editor welcomes approaches and feedback, positive and/or negative.

David has specialised in mental health and substance use for over 30 years. He has worked as a practitioner, manager, researcher, author, lecturer and consultant. He has served as editor, or editor-in-chief, of several journals, and is currently editor-in-chief of *Mental Health and Substance Use: dual diagnosis*. He has published widely and is *'credited with enhancing the understanding and development of community detoxification for people experiencing alcohol withdrawal'* (Nursing Council on Alcohol; Sigma Theta Tau International citations). Seminal work includes *Alcohol Home Detoxification and Assessment* and *Alcohol Use*, both published by Radcliffe Publishing, Oxford.

List of contributors

CHAPTER 2   Anne Bury
Independent Educator and Practitioner
Barnstaple, Devon, UK

Anne trained as an adult and children's nurse. She has worked in Saudi Arabia and Florida, USA, returning to London before leaving nursing to undertake a degree in Sociology, followed by a Postgraduate Certificate in Education. Anne held a position teaching sociology and social policy to undergraduates and student nurses at the University of Plymouth. During this time, she completed a master's degree in Policy and Organisations. Anne returned to her first love, palliative care, and worked as Head of Education, Dorothy House Hospice, then moved to a similar position at North Devon Hospice. She now works as an independent consultant, educator and practitioner.

CHAPTER 3   Professor Phil Barker
Honorary Professor
Faculty of Medicine, Dentistry, and Nursing, University of Dundee
Psychotherapist
Newport-on-Tay, Fife, UK

Phil is a psychotherapist and Honorary Professor in the School of Medicine, Dentistry and Nursing, University of Dundee. He was: the UK's first Professor of Psychiatric Nursing Practice at the University of Newcastle (1993–2002); elected a Fellow of the Royal College of Nursing in 1995; awarded the Red Gate Award for Distinguished Professors at the University of Tokyo in 2000; awarded an honorary doctorate of the University at Oxford Brookes University in 2001; and has been Visiting Professor at several international universities. In 2008 Phil (along with Poppy Buchanan-Barker) received the Thomas S. Szasz Award for Outstanding Contributions to the Cause of Civil Liberties.

CHAPTER 4   Dr Caroline O'Grady
Advanced Practice Nurse
Project Scientist
Adjunct Professor
Graduate Department of Nursing Science, University of Toronto
Concurrent Disorders Service
The Centre for Addiction and Mental Health, Toronto, Canada

Caroline is an Advanced Practice Nurse and Clinical Project Scientist in the Concurrent Disorders Service at the Centre for Addiction and Mental Health (CAMH). Since 2001, Caroline has been the lead investigator of the first Canadian programme of research focusing on family members affected by co-occurring mental health and substance use disorders. She was the Principal Investigator of a very successful innovative new research study piloting a 12-week professionally facilitated online family concurrent disorders peer support/educational group. In addition, Caroline is evaluating an Ontario-wide family concurrent disorders community of practice initiative. Caroline co-authored the book *A Family Guide to Concurrent Disorders*, and is an adjunct professor and an associate member of the University of Toronto Graduate Department of Nursing Science.

CHAPTER 5 Professor Charlotte de Crespigny (*also* Chapter 14)
Professor of Drug and Alcohol Nursing
Joint Chair and Fellow, RCNA
Discipline of Nursing
University of Adelaide Drug and Alcohol Services South Australia
Netherby, South Australia, Australia

Charlotte is a registered nurse who has worked in the drug and alcohol field as a clinician, educator and researcher since 1988. She is currently Joint Chair, Professor of Drug and Alcohol Nursing, Discipline of Nursing, The University of Adelaide and Drug and Alcohol Services, South Australia (DASSA). Charlotte works in partnership with other researchers and practitioners from acute care, mental health, public health, health economics and Aboriginal health. She is committed to translating research findings into everyday healthcare, including clinical practice, health promotion, and community and professional education. She works from the primary healthcare paradigm, particularly in relation to understanding and responding to the social, economic and environmental determinants of health, ill health and drug and alcohol problems. Charlotte is a life member of Drug and Alcohol Nurses of Australasia.

Peter Athanasos (*also* Chapter 14)
Lecturer
Coordinator of Addiction and Mental Health Programs
Discipline of Nursing
Royal Adelaide Hospital
University of Adelaide
Adelaide, South Australia, Australia

Peter is a Lecturer and the Coordinator of Addiction and Mental Health Programmes at the University of Adelaide. Peter's area of greatest research interest is the effect of substance use on coexisting disorders, such as mental health, pain and other pathophysiology. He has published on addiction, acute and chronic pain, opioid detoxification, opioid withdrawal hyperalgesia, vasodepressor syncope, cardiac effects of opioid dependency and the effects of opioid and non-opioid analgesics in opioid maintained subjects. He has also authored a textbook on addiction and chapters on mood disorders, effects of heat waves, human rights, and acute and chronic pain in the context of opioid use.

Jacky Talmet
Regional Manager
Clinical Services Coordinator Central/Country Services
Drug and Alcohol Services South Australia Inner City
Country Community Services
Adelaide, South Australia, Australia

Jacky has expertise as a specialist drug and alcohol nurse with a strong mental and community health background. For the last 25 years, she has worked as Regional Manager/ Clinical Services and Coordinator Country Community Services for Drug and Alcohol Services. More recently, she has assumed the role of manager of DASSA Central Adelaide Services. Jacky has a Master of Public Health and plays an important role supporting clinicians and educators involved in health promotion and community development in relation to prevention and treatment of alcohol, tobacco and other drug problems. She is a strong advocate of upholding the right of people to receive equitable quality health services and to responding effectively to nurses with ATOD problems. Jacky has an interest in the impact of young people's ATOD issues on families and the supports they require, and the impact of homelessness on people with ATOD and mental health issues.

Dr Anne Wilson
Senior Lecturer
Discipline of Nursing
School of Population Health and Clinical Practice
University of Adelaide
Adelaide, South Australia, Australia

Anne is an experienced community health clinician and educator with a special interest in health promotion. She has an extensive background in hospital and community nursing encompassing adults, youth and children. Anne has worked in multidisciplinary health teams as either team member or leader. Her research focuses on health services, advanced nursing practice initiatives and prevention of chronic illness. She conducted a major review of the needs of families, and others bereaved through suicide, and many of the recommendations of her work have been implemented nationally in practice and policy. Anne leads the research cluster *Changing Workforce* in the Discipline of Nursing, University of Adelaide.

Janice Elliott
Clinical Lecturer
Discipline of Nursing
The University of Adelaide
Adelaide, South Australia, Australia

Janice has worked specifically in the Emergency setting since the 1990s. Her roles included clinician, clinical leader and manager. Since 2009, she has been a lecturer and coordinator of the Postgraduate Diploma in Nursing Science (Emergency Nursing). Janice has witnessed many changes within the health setting, including the transition of emergency mental healthcare from psychiatric hospitals to the general hospital setting. She participated in the National Institute of Clinical Studies Community of Practice and Emergency Department and Mental Health Collaborative. Janice is a passionate believer in the rights of all people to receive a safe standard of care, delivered by non-judgemental, skilled clinicians within the most appropriate environment.

CHAPTER 6   Dr John R Ashcroft
Associate Specialist Psychiatrist, Substance Use
Lancashire Care Foundation Trust
Preston, Lancashire, UK

John is an Associate Specialist Psychiatrist in Substance Misuse. He studied at Imperial College of Science Technology and Medicine in London and achieved undergraduate degrees of BSc (Hons) in Neurosciences and Medicine (MBBS). He is a Member of the Royal College of Psychiatrists. In 2008, John was awarded a Postgraduate Diploma in Clinical Neuropsychiatry with merit by the University of Birmingham. He has recently been invited to become an advisory board member of the journal *Mental Health and Substance Use: dual diagnosis* published by Taylor and Francis International. He has specialist interests in clinical neuropsychiatry and dual diagnosis.

CHAPTER 7   Carol Kirby
Senior Lecturer
School of Nursing
University of Ulster at Magee
Derry, Northern Ireland

Carol is a Senior Lecturer at the University of Ulster in Northern Ireland, where she is involved in nurse education and research, primarily within the mental health and healthcare ethics contexts. She previously worked extensively in clinical practice and education, holding senior management appointments in both. Carol has produced a number of academic publications and presented papers at both national and international conferences. She is currently completing a PhD on the illness experience.

Dr Oliver D Slevin
Lecturer
Course Director, Professional Doctorate and MSc
School of Nursing
University of Ulster at Jordanstown
Newtownabbey, Northern Ireland

Oliver is a Lecturer at the University of Ulster in Northern Ireland, where he is involved in healthcare education, research and international development work through the University's Health Research & Development Group. He held a number of clinical and educational posts across Northern Ireland, Scotland and England. Previously, he was Chief Executive of the National Board for Nursing, Midwifery and Health Visiting in Northern Ireland and Associate Professor at the University of Ulster. Oliver undertook his PhD at Queen's University Belfast and has produced a large number of publications and conference presentations.

CHAPTER 8 Dr Alyna Turner
Heart Research Centre
North Melbourne
Victoria, Australia

Alyna is a clinical psychologist who has practised in liaison psychiatry, psychiatric reha-bilitation and community chronic illness services over the last 11 years. She has held a Postdoctoral Research Fellow position at the University of Newcastle and is currently Senior Research Fellow at the Heart Research Centre in Melbourne. She has contributed to trials evaluating integrated psychological treatment for mental health–substance use problems, in addition to research into assessment and treatment of mental health problems in people with chronic physical illness.

Professor Amanda L Baker
Faculty of Health
Centre for Brain and Mental Health Research
University of Newcastle
Callaghan, New South Wales, Australia

Amanda is a clinical psychologist who has practised in both mental health and alcohol and other drug treatment settings in the UK and Australia. She is currently an NHMRC Senior Research Fellowship holder at the University of Newcastle, Australia. Amanda has specialised in the treatment of mental health–substance use problems. She has led numerous trials funded by competitive national grants investigating integrated psycho-logical treatments for these problems, and has published widely in the field.

CHAPTER 9 Professor Kim T Mueser
Psychiatry, and Community and Family Medicine
Dartmouth Medical School
Concord, New Hampshire, USA

Kim is a clinical psychologist and a Professor of Psychiatry and of Community and Family Medicine at the Dartmouth Medical School. He received his PhD in psychology from the University of Illinois at Chicago in 1984, and then joined the faculty of the Psychiatry Department at Drexel University College of Medicine in Philadelphia. In 1994, he moved to Dartmouth. Kim's clinical and research interests include the psychi-atric rehabilitation of schizophrenia and other severe mental illnesses. He has published numerous articles, chapters and books, and has given numerous lectures and workshops nationally and internationally.

CHAPTER 10 Dr Carmel Clancy
Principal Lecturer, Mental Health and Substance Uses
Member, Advisory Council of the Misuse of Drugs

Department of Mental Health and Social Work
School of Health and Social Sciences
Middlesex University, London, UK

Carmel has worked in the field of mental health for approximately 25 years, with the majority of her direct clinical, managerial, teaching and research activities focused in the area of addiction. She is currently employed as a Principal Lecturer in mental health and addictions, and is Director of Programmes for the Department of Mental Health and Social Work. Until recently, she was programme leader for the MSc course in dual diagnosis (first in the UK). Carmel was Chairperson of the Association of Nurses in Substance Abuse for three years. She is also a member of the Advisory Council on the Misuse of Drugs.

Dr Adenekan Oyefeso
Reader
St George's Medical School University of London
London, UK

Adenekan is a reader at St George's Medical School University of London and honorary clinical psychologist in South West London and St George's Mental Health NHS Trust. He has worked in the field of mental health and addictions for over 25 years, and has published over 150 peer-reviewed articles and reports.

CHAPTER 11   Philip D Cooper
Practice Educator
Education and Workforce Development
Suffolk Mental Health Partnership NHS Trust
St Clements Hospital
Ipswich, Suffolk, UK

Phil qualified as a mental health nurse in 2002, and then worked within an acute admissions ward before moving to community mental health. After a brief spell in an Assertive Outreach Team, Phil moved to his current role. Here, Phil was seconded as Project Manager for the mental health–substance use needs assessment and strategy development project. Phil studied for an Advanced Diploma in Dual Diagnosis before completing an MSc in Dual Diagnosis, in 2007. Phil has authored a number of chapters, and was the founder, and editor, of the international journal *Mental Health and Substance Use: dual diagnosis*. He stepped down from this position in June 2010.

CHAPTER 12   Dr Cynthia MA Geppert
Chief Consultation Psychiatry and Ethics
New Mexico Veteran's Affairs Health Care System
Associate Professor and Director of Ethics Education
Department of Psychiatry
University of New Mexico
Albuquerque, New Mexico, USA

Cynthia is Chief of Consultation Psychiatry and Ethics at the New Mexico Veterans Affairs Health Care System, Associate Professor in the Department of Psychiatry, and Director of Ethics Education at the University of New Mexico School of Medicine. She is board certified in general psychiatry, psychosomatic medicine, and hospice and palliative medicine, certified by the American board of Addiction Medicine and holds credentials in pain management. She specialises in the treatment of patients with medical illnesses, co-occurring disorders, chronic pain and in palliative care. Cynthia teaches, writes and conducts research in the fields of consultation psychiatry, clinical ethics, spirituality, medical education, addiction and psychopharmacology.

CHAPTER 13   Dr Chris Holmwood
Senior Consultant
Clinical Services and Research
Drug and Alcohol Services South Australia
Norwood, South Australia, Australia

Chris is currently Director, Clinical Workforce Development and Standards for Drug and Alcohol Services South Australia. He has a background in general practice and for five years was the Director of the South Australian Prison Health Service. He has particular clinical interests in the care of people with complex comorbidities, pain and substance dependence, as well as medical education and chronic disease management.

CHAPTER 14   Dr Lynette Cusack
Research Fellow (Population Health)
School of Nursing and Midwifery
Faculty of Health Science
Flinders University
Adelaide, South Australia, Australia

Lynette works with Professor P Arbon in the area of population health, specialising in the preparedness, response, recovery and development of communities related to disaster management. The focus in relation to disaster management is on community development, impact of heatwaves on vulnerable groups within the population, support to aged care facilities preparing for emergency events/disasters and evacuation. Lynette has worked in the alcohol and other drug field as Director of Community Services, with the Drug and Alcohol Services South Australia, which is a State Government organisation.

Professor Charlotte de Crespigny (*see* Chapter 5)

Peter Athanasos (*see* Chapter 5)

USEFUL CONTACTS   Jo Cooper

Jo spent 16 years in Specialist Palliative Care, initially working in a hospice inpatient unit, then 12 years as a Macmillan Clinical Nurse Specialist. She gained a Diploma in

Oncology at Addenbrooke's Hospital, Cambridge, and a BSc (Hons) in Palliative Nursing at The Royal Marsden, London, and an Award in Specialist Practice. Jo edited *Stepping into Palliative Care* (2000) and the 2nd edition, *Stepping into Palliative Care, Books 1 and 2* (2006), both published by Radcliffe Publishing. Jo has been involved in teaching for many years and her specialist subjects include management of complex pain and symptoms, terminal agitation, communication at the end of life, therapeutic relationships and breaking bad news.

Terminology

Whenever possible, the following terminology has been applied. However, in certain instances, when referencing a study and/or specific work(s), when an author has made a specific request, or for the purpose of additional clarity, it has been necessary to deviate from this applied 'norm'.

MENTAL HEALTH–SUBSTANCE USE

Considerable thought has gone in to the use of terminology within these texts. Each country appears to have its own terms for the person experiencing a mental health and substance use problem – terms that includes words such as dual diagnosis, coexisting, co-occurring, and so on. We talk about the same thing but use differing professional jargon. The decision was set at the outset to use one term that encompasses mental health *and* substance use problems: *mental health–substance use*. One scholar suggested that such a term implies that both can exist separately, while they can also be linked.[1]

SUBSTANCE USE

Another challenge was how to term 'substance use'. There are a number of ways: abuse, misuse, dependence, addiction. The decision is that within these texts we use the term *substance use* to encompass all (unless specific need for clarity at a given point). It is imperative the professional recognises that while we may see another person's 'substance use' as misuse or abuse, the individual experiencing it may not deem it to be anything other than 'use'. Throughout, we need to be aware that we are working alongside unique individuals. Therefore, we should be able to meet the individual where he/she is.

ALCOHOL, PRESCRIBED DRUGS, ILLICIT DRUGS, TOBACCO OR SUBSTANCE

Throughout this book *substance* includes *alcohol*, *prescribed drugs*, *illicit drugs* and *tobacco*, unless specific need for clarity at a given point.

PROBLEM(S), CONCERNS AND DILEMMAS OR DISORDERS

The terms *problem(s)*, *concerns and dilemmas* and *disorders* can be used interchangeably, as stated by the author's preference. However, where possible, the term 'problem(s)' or 'concerns and dilemmas' had been adopted as the preferred choice.

INDIVIDUAL, PERSON, PEOPLE

There seems to be a need to label the individual – as a form of recognition! Sometimes the label becomes more than the person! 'Alan is schizophrenic' – thus it is Alan, rather than an illness that Alan lives with. We refer to patients, clients, service users, customers, consumers, and so on. Yet, we feel affronted when we are addressed as anything other than what we are – individuals! We need to be mindful that every person we see during our professional day is an individual – unique. Symptoms are in many ways similar (e.g. delusions, hallucinations) and some require intervention; treatments are also similar (e.g. specific drugs, psychotherapy techniques), *but* people are not. Alan may experience an illness labelled schizophrenia, and so may John, Beth and Mary, and you or me. However, each will have his/her own unique experiences – and life. None will be the same. To keep this constantly in the mind of the reader, throughout the book series we shall refer to the *individual*, *person* or *people* – just like us, but different to us by their uniqueness.

PROFESSIONAL

We are all professionals, whether students, nurses, doctors, social workers, researchers, clinicians, educationalist, managers, service developers, religious ministers – and so on. However, the level of expertise may vary from one professional to another. We are also individuals. There is a need to distinguish between the person with a mental health–substance use problem and the person interacting professionally (at whatever level) with that individual. To acknowledge and to differentiate between those who experience – in this context – and those who intervene, we have adopted the term *professional*. It is indicative that we have had, or are receiving, education and training related specifically to help us (the professionals) meet the needs of the individual. We may or may not have experienced mental health–substance use problems but we have some knowledge that may help the individual – an expertise to be shared. We have a specific knowledge that, hopefully, we wish to use to offer effective intervention and treatment to another human being. It is the need to make a clear differential, for the reader, that forces the use of 'professional' over 'individual' to describe our role – our input into another person's life.

REFERENCE

1 Barker P. Personal communication; 2009.

Cautionary note

*Wisdom and compassion should become the dominating influence that guide our
thoughts, our words, and our actions.*[1]

Never presume that what you say is understood. It is essential to check understanding,
and what is expected of the individual and/or family, with each person. Each person
needs to know what he/she can expect from you, and other professionals involved in his/
her care, at each meeting. Jargon is a professional language that excludes the individual
and family. Never use it in conversation with the individual, unless requested to do so;
it is easily misunderstood.

Remember, we all, as individuals, deal with life differently. It does not matter how
many years we have spent studying human behaviour, listening and treating the individual and family. We may have spent many hours exploring with the individual his/
her anxieties, fears, doubts, concerns and dilemmas, and the illness experience. Yet, we
do not know what that person really feels, how he/she sees life and ill health. We may
have lived similar lives, experienced the same illness but the individual will always be
unique, each different from us, each independent of our thoughts, feelings, words, deeds
and symptoms, each with an individual experience.

REFERENCE
1 Matthieu Ricard. As cited in: Föllmi D, Föllmi O. *Buddhist Offerings 365 Days*. London: Thames
   and Hudson; 2003.

Acknowledgements

I am grateful to all the contributors for having the faith in me to produce a valued text and I thank them for their support and encouragement. I hope that faith proves correct. Thank you to those who have commented along the way, and whose patience has been outstanding. Thank you to Jo Cooper, who has been actively involved with this project throughout – supporting, encouraging, listening and participating in many practical ways. Jo is my rock who looks after me during my physical health problems, and I am eternally grateful.

Many people have helped me along my career path and life – too many to name individually. Most do not even know what impact they have had on me. Some, however, require specific mention. These include Larry Purnell, a friend and confidant who has taught me never to presume – while we are all individuals with individual needs, we deserve equality in all that we meet in life. Thanks to Martin Plant (who sadly died in March 2010), and Moira Plant, who always encouraged and offered genuine support. Phil and Poppy Barker, who have taught me that it is OK to express how I feel about humanity – about people, and that there is another way through the entrenched systems in health and social care. Keith Yoxhall, without whose guidance back in the 1980s I would never have survived my 'Colchester work experience' and the dark times of institutionalisation, or had the privilege to work alongside the few professionals fighting against the 'big door'. He taught me that there was a need for education and training, and that this should be ongoing – also that the person in hospital or community experiencing our care sees us a 'professional' – we should make sure we act that way. Thank you to Phil Cooper, who brought the concept of this book series to me via a conference to launch the journal *Mental Health and Substance Use: dual diagnosis*, of which he was editor. It was then I realised that despite all the talk over too many years of my professional life, there was still much to be done for people experiencing mental health–substance use problems. Phil is a good debater, friend and reliable resource for me – thank you.

To Gillian Nineham of Radcliffe Publishing, my sincere thanks. Gillian had faith in this project from the outset and in my ability to deliver. Her patience is immeasurable and, for that, I am grateful. Thank you to Michael Hawkes for putting up with my too numerous questions! Thank you to Jamie Etherington, Editorial Development Manager, and Dan Allen of the book marketing department, both competent people who makes my work look good. Thanks also to Mia Yardley and the production team at Pindar, New Zealand, for bringing this book to publication, and the many others who are nameless to me as I write but without whom these books would never come to print; each has his/her stamp on any successes of this book.

My sincere thanks to all of you named, and unnamed, my friends and colleagues along my sometimes broken career path: those who have touched my life in a positive way – and a few, a negative way (for we can learn from the negative to ensure we do better for others).

A final heartfelt statement: any errors, omissions, inaccuracies or deficiencies within these pages are my sole responsibility.

Dedication

This book – and my life – is dedicated to Jo. A special person of unquestioning faith, trust, support, care, and love – at all times. Her encouragement makes the concepts flow to fruition, and for that, I am unreservedly thankful. Her non-judgemental caring in her professional years for the individual and family, and her total and absolute, non-judgemental care for our children and grandchildren is immeasurable.

  . . . and when my courage fails me, I shall think of you – and hold fast.[1]

Reference

1 Thompson F. *Lark Rise to Candleford: a trilogy*. London: Penguin Modern Classics; 2009.

CHAPTER 1

Setting the scene

David B Cooper

It is only through constant training that our practice will grow steady and we will be able to control our negative tendencies fearlessly.[1]

PRE-READING EXERCISE 1.1

Time: 20 minutes
When preparing to read this book you may wish to undertake the following exercise.
Write a brief description of your thoughts and feelings in relation to mental health–substance use problems. When you have read the book repeat the exercise, taking note of the following.
- Have your thoughts and feelings changed? If yes, in what way?
- What information do you feel most influenced that change? What did not?
- Are there any areas that you feel you need to investigate further? If yes, what are they? What resources will you need?
- Make a plan of action to develop your learning and understanding of mental health–substance use.

INTRODUCTION

The difficulties encountered by people who experience mental health–substance use problems are not new. The individual using substances presenting to the mental health professional can often encounter annoyance and suspicion. Likewise, the person experiencing mental health problems presenting to the substance use services can encounter hostility and hopelessness. 'We cannot do anything for the substance use problem until the mental health problem is dealt with!' The referral to the mental health team is returned: 'We cannot do anything for this person until the substance use problem is dealt with!' Thus, the individual is in the middle of two professional worlds and neither is willing to move, and yet, both professional worlds are involved in 'caring' for the individual.

For many years, it has been acknowledged that the two parts of the caring system need to work as one. However, this desire has not developed into practice. Over recent years, this impetus has changed. There is now a drive towards meeting the needs of the

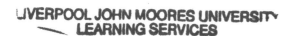

individual experiencing mental health–substance use problems, pooling expertise from both sides. Moreover, there is an international political will to bring about change, often driven forward by a small group of dedicated professionals at practice level.

Some healthcare environments have merely paid lip service, ensuring the correct terminology is included within the policy and procedure documentation, while at the same time doing nothing, or little, to bring about the changes needed at the practice level to meet the needs of the individual. Others have grasped the drive forward and have spearheaded developments at local and national level within their country to meet such needs. It appears that the latter are now succeeding. There is a concerted international effort to improve the services provided for the individual, and a determination to pool knowledge and expertise. In addition, there is the ability of these professional groups to link into government policy and bring about the political will to support such change. However, this cannot happen overnight. There are major attitudinal changes needed – not least at management and practice level. One consultant commented that to work together with mental health–substance use problems would be too costly. Furthermore, the consultant believed it would create 'too much work'! Consequently, there is a long way to go – but a driving force to succeed exists.

Obtaining in-depth and knowledgeable text is difficult in new areas of change. One needs to be motivated to trawl a broad spectrum of work to develop a sound grounding – the background detail that is needed to build good professional practice. This is a big request of the hard-worked and pressured professional. There are a few excellent mental health–substance use books available. However, this series of six books, of which this is the first, is ground-breaking, in that each presents a much-needed text that will introduce the first, but vital, step to the interventions and treatments available for the individual experiencing mental health–substance use concerns and dilemmas.

These books are educational. However, they will make no one an expert! In mental health–substance use, there is a need to initiate, and maintain, education and training. There are key principles and factors we need to bring out and explore. Some we will use – others we will adapt – while others we will reject. Each book is complete. Conversely, each aims to build on the preceding book. However, books *do not* hold all the answers. Nothing does. What is hoped is that the professional will participate in, and collaborate with, each book, progressing through each to the other. Along the way, hopefully, the professional will enhance existing knowledge or develop new concepts to benefit the individual.

The books offer a first step, relevant to the needs of professionals – at practice level or senior service development – in a clear, concise and understandable format. Each book has made full use of boxes, graphs, tables, figures, interactive exercises, self-assessment tools and case studies – where appropriate – to examine and demonstrate the effect mental health–substance use can have on the individual, family, carers and society as a whole.

A deliberate attempt has been made to avoid jargon, and where terminology is used, to offer a clear explanation and understanding. The terminology used in this book is fully explained at the beginning of each book, before the reader commences with the chapters. By placing it there the reader will be able to reference it quickly, if needed. Specific gender is used, as the author feels appropriate. However, unless stated, the use of the male/female gender is interchangeable.

BOOK 1: INTRODUCTION TO MENTAL HEALTH–SUBSTANCE USE

The analogy of the house purchaser sums up the approach of the editor and authors when writing this book. Once a property is identified, we need to find out more before we invest further – the first step is to visit the property. On arrival we quickly grasp a view of the surrounding area, the look of the outside of the house and its grounds. Here we make the decision to enter the property to find out more – or we leave. It is hoped that the reader of this book will stay! The book takes the reader through the front door of mental health–substance use, for some that will be all that is needed, for a decision to be made, and they will proceed to *own the property*. Others will need more information or guidance on the many and diverse approaches to mental health–substance use.

We can never know all there is to know. There is always the need to remain open-minded in the approaches to the individual's needs and expectations. It is essential that we are open-minded to the many differing ways we can bring about change, and how we can access new information and knowledge. This applies in terms of both self-learning, and the way we approach interventions with those who are in need of advice and guidance. Each chapter provides direction to further learning and exploration.

Many learned professionals are willing to share what they know and listen to the knowledge and advice of others. It is hoped that this fundamental introduction will stimulate us to 'open the door' to those in need of therapeutic interventions and treatments resulting from problems related to their, or someone else's, experiences of mental health–substance use.

As mentioned in the preface, the ability to learn and gain new knowledge is the way forward. As professionals we must start with knowledge, and from there we can begin to understand. We commence using our new-found skills, progressing to developing the ability to examine practice, to put concepts together and to make valid judgements.[2] This knowledge is gained through education, training and experience, sometimes enhanced by own life experiences.

Those we offer care to, and their family members, also bring their own knowledge, skills and life experiences, some developed from dealing with ill health. Therefore, in order to make interventions and treatment outcome effective requires mutual understanding and respect.

In the book, primarily we:

➤ explore the comprehensive concerns and dilemmas occurring from, and in, mental health–substance use

➤ inform, develop and educate by sharing knowledge and enhancing expertise in this fast-developing interrelated experience of psychological, physical, social, legal and spiritual need.

Chapter 2 aims to introduce the unfamiliar reader to ways of learning and developing educational skills, not to be a teacher or educator but to apply learning to the professional's own experience. Following chapters build on this theme. We explore the terminology – the basis of this book and the series – and approaches to mental health–substance use. Then we look at the world of the individual who has experienced the negative consequences of the divided approach to mental health and substance use. Here we get a true feeling of what it is really like to be on the 'receiving end'.

It is correct that we explore the individuals' human rights, and the importance and impact of the mental health and substance use experience. However, we equally need to give attention to the physical consequences, and health, of the individual. A robust, ongoing, physical health assessment is essential and should be integral to any mental health–substance use assessment. From here, we develop an understanding of the experiences of illness, of stigmatisation and the psychological impact of serious illness on the individual, family and carers, with a view to exploring the world of the individual.

Chapter 9 progresses to working with the individual, while Chapter 10 takes an in-depth look at the professional skills and capabilities needed. Chapter 11 explains the methods adopted within the Suffolk Mental Health Partnership National Health Service Trust to deal with the practical approaches to attitudes and brief training intervention. Current approaches produce many ethical concerns and Chapter 12 explores ethics and ethical dilemmas associated with mental health–substance use.

The last two chapters serve to open our mind to the fact that mental health–substance use excludes nothing and no one. We need to be aware of the environmental influences of those we care for, and that physical health and problems are interlinked and integral to mental health–substance use, and they should not be excluded or ignored.

CONCLUSION

Referring to the house analogy above, it is hoped that this introduction is helpful and informative. One would hope that we feel sufficiently stimulated to proceed, having extended and developed this grounding in mental health–substance use. Now that the basics have been explored, we can build upon our knowledge using the 'To learn more' section in each chapter as a guide to further study and knowledge. As one enters each new area of knowledge (each new room), so understanding improves. With that comes the ability to use an open, non-judgemental and accepting approach to the problems identified by the individual presenting for intervention, treatment, advice or guidance.

Our knowledge and understanding constantly change. The challenge is to remain open and accessible to the knowledge and information that will help each of us provide appropriate therapeutic interventions:
➤ at the appropriate level of expertise
➤ at the appropriate time
➤ at the appropriate level of understanding of the individual, and her/his presenting concerns and dilemmas
➤ at the appropriate cost.

We cannot afford to be cocooned in our belief that all individuals are the same. If this book encourages us to learn more, it has achieved its aim. If it helps us to appreciate some of the problems encountered by the individual, family and carers, it has 'opened the door'.

To see the preciousness of all things, we must bring our full attention to life.[3]

REFERENCES

1 Dilgo Khyentse Rinpoche. As cited in: Föllmi D, Föllmi O. *Buddhist Offerings 365 Days*. London: Thames and Hudson; 2003.

2 Bloom BS, Hastings T, Madaus G. *Handbook of Formative and Summative Evaluation*. New York, NY: McGraw-Hill; 1971.

3 Jack Kornfield. As cited in: Föllmi D, Föllmi O. *Buddhist Offerings 365 Days*. London: Thames and Hudson; 2003.

CHAPTER 2

Learning to learn

Anne Bury

Any healer is only as good as his ability to heal himself, any teacher can only teach that which he already inwardly knows.[1]

PRE-READING EXERCISE 2.1

Time: 30 minutes
1   What do you think is necessary to provide good care for people with mental health–substance use concerns and dilemmas?
2   Think of a time when you were either an individual or family. Remember a health professional that you felt *really understood* and *connected with* your needs.
   • What was it about this person, what knowledge, skills and qualities did he/she have?
   • How do you think he/she learnt them?
3   Now, think back to the first person you offered professional intervention and treatment to who you felt emotionally touched by, either someone you were close to, or someone who made you feel angry.
   • What sticks out in your mind?
   • What support was offered to that person, the family and yourself?
   • Did you feel emotionally and practically prepared?
   • What education and training had you received?
   • What knowledge do you think you needed?

HOW DO WE LEARN?

Being an effective practitioner involves learning both the art and science of healthcare. While the emphasis in undergraduate education may have been on the technical and scientific aspects of care, learning to be an effective professional is more than that. People with mental health–substance use problems inevitably struggle with deep spiritual distress and soul pain and are recognised as one of the most vulnerable groups in society.[2] Therefore, the individual needs the professional to be alongside. Relating as one human being to another requires each professional to learn the art of connecting, as whole person to whole person, soul to soul. This can present us with a challenge, given

the increasing emphasis on:
➤ measurement
➤ targets
➤ outcomes
➤ the medicalisation of mental healthcare
➤ the social construction
➤ the stigmatisation of the individual
➤ the way the individual and family may put up barriers to meaningful communication.

As you read this chapter, imagine that you are going on a journey. You will be wearing special rose-coloured lenses to help challenge and question your:
➤ self
➤ understanding of mental health–substance use care
➤ education, training and learning.

Take the time to reflect on what you already know and consider important. Explore your own:
➤ feelings: how does this work make you feel?
➤ values: what is important to you?
➤ attitudes: in what ways may you judge the individual and family – consciously and unconsciously?
➤ experience: what is your own experience of mental health–substance use?

Consider:
➤ how you learn
➤ from whom you learn
➤ what stops you learning
➤ what you need to unlearn.

SO WHY DO YOU NEED TO LEARN?
There are higher levels of depressive, affective problems, schizophrenia and personality disorders among those with substance use problems.[3] Media, and health professionals, often focus on the negative impact of mental health–substance use. There is a tendency to blame the individual, or family, rather than explore the underlying societal and cultural reasons why people may experience mental health–substance use problems. Alcohol in particular is commonly accepted and embedded within our culture and people's lifestyles. Mental health and substance use are linked to a complex and interactive array of psychological, social, economic, legal and environmental factors.[4] Therefore, working with the individual and family with mental health–substance use problems inevitably requires you to look beyond the 'individual', taking account of the 'whole'.

Recently, healthcare policy and practice have identified the interrelated and interdependent relationship between mental health and substance use. This has gradually been recognised in service provision, in some small way, although integrated services remain scarce.[3]

With the above information in mind, we need to reflect upon:
➤ what we know
➤ what education we have received
➤ our understanding, attitudes and experience
➤ how we can learn to care more effectively, for the individual – as a whole.

KEY AREAS OF KNOWLEDGE IN MENTAL HEALTHCARE

The practice of mental health–substance use care is an art and science. They are intertwined; both are essential. However, over recent years scientific knowledge and technical aspects, such as symptom management and outcome measurement, have received greater legitimacy and emphasis.[5]

Seminal research[6] into the breadth of knowledge required in palliative care has value and significance for mental health–substance use care, most of which is linked to the art of care (*see* Figure 2.1).

The *three kinds of knowing* (*see* Box 2.1)[7] and *four patterns of knowing* (*see* Box 2.2)[8] provide useful frameworks to explore the different types of knowledge base required. Each is important in its own right. However, they overlap and are interrelated.

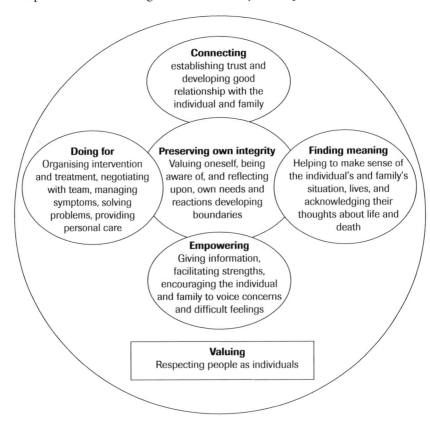

FIGURE 2.1 Adapted dimensions of supportive role (Davies and Oberle)[6]

BOX 2.1 Three kinds of knowing (Habermas)[7]

1 *Instrumental/technical knowing* – acquisition of skills and understanding.
2 *Communicative knowing* – interpersonal relations, social and cultural understanding.
3 *Emancipatory knowing* – self-understanding, awareness and transformation.

BOX 2.2 Four patterns of knowing (Carper)[8]

1 *Empirics* – based on a scientific evidence-based approach and can be seen as *know that* knowledge. This includes objective knowledge about the disease process, technical knowledge, symptom management and interventions based on an evidence base.
2 *Ethical* – awareness and understanding of ethical, moral and professional issues, notions of right or wrong. This area is integral in all decision making and underpins professional judgement.
3 *Personal* – based on gaining self-mastery, becoming self-aware and self-reflective. This personal knowing is at the heart of our ability to care for others and the development of a therapeutic relationship (*see* Book 4, Chapter 2). We need to have compassion for ourselves; we need, as professionals, to be our own carers first. If we can learn to sit with and understand our own pain, anger or fear, have compassion and forgive ourselves, we are more likely to be there for the individual and his/her family.
4 *Aesthetic* – based on intuition and intuitive learning and is considered to be the art and *know how* of nursing. Intuition enables people to respond to things creatively using imagination and abstract thinking. It is this knowledge that enables us to have *an intuitive grasp*. We are able to know what to do. We know that something is right or recognise a change in someone's condition without consciously knowing why. When we try to describe aesthetic knowledge we often find ourselves lost for words. This can be seen as tacit knowledge.

NOVICE TO EXPERT

We need to evolve from being novice to expert professional. As novices, we need to be taught technical and rule-based knowledge and do things *by the book*. As experts, we need to be able to unconsciously utilise and incorporate all the above knowledge and develop our '*intuitive grasp*'. To be *expert*, we cannot solely rely on our art, we need to test out and challenge our theory-based knowledge in practice, and to systematically record and reflect upon our practice-based knowledge. Only through this can expertise be achieved. We develop expertise through:

➤ interpreting clinical situations
➤ exploring and critiquing the evidence
➤ making complex decisions.

Therefore, knowledge is embedded in clinical expertise.[9]

SELF-ASSESSMENT EXERCISE 2.1

Time: 20 minutes
Consider how you might use:
- Davies and Oberle's aspects[6]
- Carper's ways of knowing[8]
- Benner's concept of novice to expert[9]

as a framework for intervention and treatment for the individual and family.

Identify:
- where you think you are on the novice–expert continuum
- what you know from theory and practice
- what your learning needs are.

Consider:
- how you learnt your knowledge
- how you might meet your learning needs.

SO HOW DO WE LEARN THIS KNOWLEDGE?

Lifelong learning has been recognised as important.[10] Continuing professional development is imperative for all professionals to enable them to demonstrate their competence to practise. Importantly, formal and informal learning are recognised as of equal value. Learning from practice and experience is viewed as essential.

Competences and areas of need[11] have been identified and include the following.

1 Off-job learning and development with others.
2 On-job learning and development.
3 Off-job learning and development on one's own.

Figure 2.2 provides a summary of what we need to consider, and include, when learning about mental healthcare–substance use.

1 Off-job learning and development with others: classroom-based learning

Traditionally, learning has been seen as formal, taking place in the classroom and during one's youth. It has been viewed as something the teacher did to a learner. Teachers, *who were more knowledgeable*, imparted information to *those who knew less*. This form of learning is derived from a didactic approach. Those advocating an experiential approach challenge this approach. They argue that for learning to take place, learners need to be active, and process, interpret and make sense of what is presented to them. These paradigms are not opposed to each other but are at opposite ends of the spectrum; both have their place. Traditional or didactic programmes highlight knowledge and information, whereas experiential programmes encourage self-direction, reflection and involvement (*see* Table 2.1).[12]

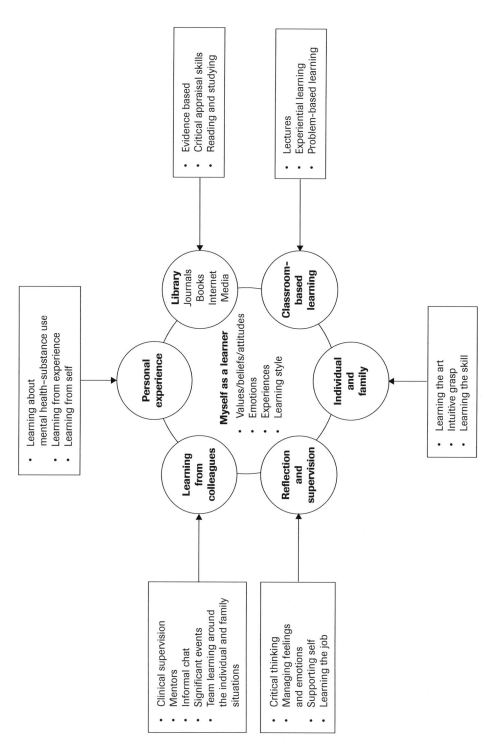

FIGURE 2.2 Learning to learn

TABLE 2.1 Distinctions between the two kinds of learning[12]

Significant experiential learning	Traditional conventional learning
Personal involvement	Prescribed curriculum
Whole person	Similar for all students
Self-initiated	Lecturing
Pervasive	Standardised testing
Evaluated by learner	Instructor evaluated
Essence is meaning	Essence is knowing and reproducing

Despite the recognition of the effectiveness of an active experiential approach to learning, the formal, more traditional, didactic lecture style is still predominant in healthcare education and training, providing little opportunity for debate, discussion, or personal sharing and learning.

Adults need more self-directed learning, with the teacher being a guide and facilitator, utilising their expertise to stimulate learning rather than to communicate a body of knowledge.[13] The key is not so much to consider *what* you are learning but *how* you are learning. Even in traditional lecture sessions, you can enhance your learning through questioning *what is being said* and relating it to *your own experience*, rather than just taking notes to be put aside once the lecture is over.

SELF-ASSESSMENT EXERCISE 2.2

Time: 5 minutes
Think about the last course/study day you attended.
● What was the topic?
● Which model of learning was being used?

As learners, you need to be aware and questioning of how you are taught.
➤ Are you involved in the learning?
➤ Are you encouraged to reflect, process and apply knowledge to experience?

Even when you are learning, something you consider to be technical and straightforward, for example, symptom management, the lecture approach is not sufficient. It may provide you with information but will not assist you in applying it to practice. The true complexity of symptom management needs to encompass all of the *domains of knowledge* and teaching strategies need to consider the three learning domains:
➤ **cognitive**: thinking, making sense, questioning – lecture, case studies
➤ **affective**: exploring our attitudes and emotions – self-reflection
➤ **psychomotor**: doing, skills development – learning through experience.[14]

Research demonstrates that the more we are involved in the learning process the more we learn (*see* Figure 2.3), and gives credence to the old Chinese proverb:

I hear and I forget
I see and I remember
I do and I understand.

The Learning Pyramid (*see* Figure 2.3), further illustrates this point. Only 5% of information received from listening in a didactic session is likely to be retained, whereas when we are allowed to learn through 'doing' the retention rate goes up to 75%.

Learning styles and whole brain thinking
People have different learning styles,[15,16] and are either right-brain or left-brain thinkers.[17] Left-brain thinking tends to be logical and systematic whereas right-brain thinking sees the big picture and is creative and intuitive. For learning to be effective, you will need to become confident with different learning styles and develop whole brain thinking.

SELF-ASSESSMENT EXERCISE 2.3

> **Time: 30 minutes**
> Consider Honey and Munford's[16] *Learning Styles Questionnaire.*
> • Are you an activist, reflector, theorist or pragmatist?
> • Are you a right- or left-brain thinker – or both?

Experiential learning
Experiential learning is the most effective form of learning. Experiential learning means learning from:
➤ current or past experience through sharing and reflecting upon your own experiences
➤ artificially created experiences; these may involve:
— role-play
— scenario-based learning
— creative approaches.

Experiential learning requires you, as the learner, to place your whole self in the situation: to develop critical and self-awareness. This can be daunting for those unused to this form of learning, believing that they are there to learn – and the teacher is there to teach.

Hearing the voice
Have you attended an education and teaching session in which an individual or family member has recalled his/her story, and shared what it is like to be the recipient of mental health–substance use intervention and treatment? It helps to put ourselves in others' shoes, which can be very difficult when someone is angry or distressed. Although you engage with the individual every day, actually sitting down and hearing *how it is*, in a classroom situation, can be challenging and upsetting. Moreover, it can make us think about our own personal experiences.

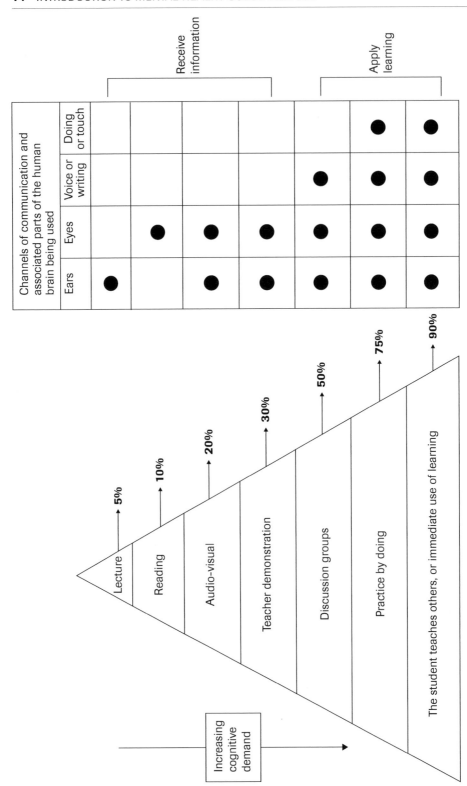

FIGURE 2.3 *The Learning Pyramid.* Source: *Research on the recall rate of different learning activities* (National Training Laboratories, Bethel, Maine, USA)

SELF-ASSESSMENT EXERCISE 2.4

Time: 30 minutes
Read the following stories. Note down your initial reactions to them and identify the relationship between this and their mental and emotional health.
- Note down your own personal experiences of mental health–substance use.
- How old were you when you had your first experience.
- Did you use substances to self-medicate? In what way?
- Are there ways in which you can identify with the three people in these stories?
- Note these down and reflect upon reasons why your use has not spiralled out of control.
- Have you had experience of family members or friends with mental health–substance use concerns and dilemmas?
- What was the impact on them and on yourself?
- How can you use your own experiences to help you understand that of others?

'I remember when I started drinking. I have had several bouts of depression where drink has always been involved. I tend to drink to block things out'.[3]

'I experimented with drugs a lot at university, but so did everyone. I ended a three-year relationship, and had an abortion. My father died soon after and my close friends let me down. I think I was depressed. People avoided me. I don't know why. My drug use spiralled. I hurt everybody. It taken me over, I am dead'.[3]

'I looked after my mother but I couldn't deal with the emotions without a drink. I wanted to be normal. Stop feeling anxious. My head was always full of stuff. Vodka helps me forget'[3]

Problem-based learning
A new experiential learning strategy is *problem-based learning*.[18] This student-centred approach provides a systematic interactive approach to critical thinking and clinical judgement, combined with the use of reflective journals to encourage learners to reflect in, and learn from, practice. This approach provides:
➤ increased self-awareness
➤ more positive attitudes
➤ enhanced communication in difficult situations
➤ emotional support
➤ critical thinking
➤ teamwork.

This could be a valuable approach to intra- and interdisciplinary learning in mental health–substance use interventions and treatment, enabling and enhancing:
➤ a shared understanding of each other
➤ collaboration
➤ individual and family intervention and treatment.

Learning to be a critical thinker

Critical thinking is an attitude and reasoning process involving a number of intellectual skills.[19] Critical thinking requires objective and subjective qualities. It requires the
ability to:

➤ think rationally, logically, practically and theoretically
➤ demonstrate self-awareness, creativity, sensitivity and responsiveness to others.

It requires:

➤ cognitive skills, including decision-making skills, problem-solving skills and
   intuition
➤ people to think independently, have intellectual humility, integrity, courage,
   empathy and perseverance
➤ people to distinguish intuition from prejudice.

To become a critical thinker you need to:

➤ critique evidence
➤ reflect on your experience
➤ question yourself, your behaviour, emotions, fears, responses, values, attitudes and
   assumptions.

You need to consider the impact of the wider political, social and economic context.
When working with the individual or family, think about the background in relation
to social and economic disadvantage, poverty, abuse, etc., in order to try to understand
the experience(s) from a structural and an individual perspective. Consider power differences, imbalances, ingrained rituals and practices, organisational and professional
restraints, and the impact of the care environment culture. With an open mind you
need to listen to:

➤ opposing views
➤ new ideas
➤ learning methods
➤ your own and others' feelings.

Most of all, you need to be prepared to unlearn what you think is right, and unlearn
your own views about yourself.

2 On-job learning and development: non-classroom-based learning

Learning is embedded in experience and practice. It is the heart of lifelong learning.
Although recognised by professional bodies and the UK *knowledge and skills* framework,[11] it is, even with all the funding restraints, easier to be released for a study day
than to be given time to learn in, and from, practice. Aesthetic knowledge hinges on this
form of learning. If you are motivated to evolve from novice to expert, you may have to
be proactive and challenge this.

Learning to manage feelings and emotions

Although emotional labour is an essential part of mental health–substance use intervention and treatment, it is an area often neglected in the curriculum. People develop their own coping strategies and often learn to distance themselves from difficult or painful situations,[20] thus affecting the relationship with the individual and or family. Often the person in charge sets the emotional climate. Crying, or showing emotions, is not deemed professional. If people are nurtured and supported, they are more likely to be able to give openly to others, to develop appropriate boundaries and to avoid burn-out.[21]

Working in mental health–substance use can be emotionally draining. You are often working with people experiencing physical, emotional, psychological, spiritual and legal problems. They are often not used to experiencing someone being alongside them, as one human to another, and may thus react angrily.

The individual or family may challenge us emotionally, cause us to be angry, or upset. It is not easy to be honest about negative feelings. However, it is impossible to be completely non-judgemental; some people will inevitably push our buttons. To develop self-awareness it is important to look at your emotions and reactions to people.

It is easier to forget that the professional offers intervention and treatment to dying people! Mental health–substance use often has physical consequences. These can lead to death or suicide. As human beings, we have anxieties and fears about death, and may have had personal and professional experiences of death and suicide. We may feel we have failed people who have committed suicide. Talking about dying can bring painful memories and emotions, particularly if you have felt unsupported at the time and have learnt to deal with these by *'being professional'* and moving on.

Mentors and peers are helpful in enabling the professional to manage his/her emotions. Knowing there is an opportunity to be heard, the professional learns to contain the distress until there is a time to reflect.[22] Through increased self-awareness he/she learns to create a form of *professional membrane*, retaining sensitivity to the individual and family while retaining integrity – being present but not enmeshed.[22]

SELF-ASSESSMENT EXERCISE 2.5

Time: 10 minutes
Consider:
- How do you manage your emotions?
- How did you learn to do this?
- What are your coping strategies?
- Who presses your buttons?

Learning from mentors

Mentorship and shadowing are recognised as essential in the education and training of students and the support of preceptors but are rarely used in day-to-day practice. Consider finding yourself someone who is knowledgeable and experienced that you can spend time with in practice. Identify someone with good interpersonal skills that you trust and respect. Invite them to be your mentor, to help you reflect and learn from your practice and share your emotional pain. They will need to be able to befriend, support, challenge, confront, question and coach you, and to commit to a regular period. Agree ground rules, learning objectives and a review date. Begin each session with a reflection on an incident, and then explore new understanding. Finally, develop an action plan. Use a reflective model or framework if you find this helpful.

Learning with a peer
Identify a colleague with whom you feel you can have an equal, reciprocal relationship. Invite them to act as peer support. You will both need all the qualities of a mentor. You can establish the relationship in a similar way. You may find it easier to be honest with each other but be less willing to challenge and analyse.

Reflection on practice
People often 'do' reflective practice on a course – and then stop! If you are inexperienced in reflection, it can help to use a model or cycle. Do this with a peer or mentor before sharing it with a group.[23,24] Reflect on an incident or situation, or keep a reflective journal. Developing your reflective skills takes time, practice and patience; the more you do the more expert you become. It enables you to:
➤ identify what happened
➤ note ritualistic care
➤ reflect on your evidence base
➤ explore your strengths and your feelings
➤ explore your attitudes and judgements
➤ be clearer about what you have learned, and what you might do differently in the future.

Moreover, it helps to identify learning in practice, the value of colleagues, and learning from the individual and family.

SELF-ASSESSMENT EXERCISE 2.6

Time: 30 minutes
Have you ever experienced an intuitive grasp? Identify an example and write about it. Using what, how, when and whom:
• describe the situation
• explain why you think it was an intuitive grasp
• say whether it was accurate
• say how you would explain the phenomenon now.

Learning from significant events/critical incidents: intra- and interdisciplinary learning
Significant event analysis should be a routine part of mental health–substance use intervention and treatment. Teams should meet together and reflect upon the individual, or a situation. This can be an experience that went well, or one that presented a challenge.

In challenging, ongoing situations, all professionals involved in the situation should:
➤ meet regularly
➤ share information, personal reactions and experiences
➤ discuss intervention and treatment options.

This facilitates realisation that others experience similar difficulties, that they are not alone in their distress. It enables a greater understanding of individual roles and encourages shared learning. Try to establish these within your own workplace.

Learning through keeping a reflective journal

> The journal is a space, like an eddy within a fast moving stream, where I can pause from the often hectic and reactive effort of stream life in order to reflect and see things the way they are.[24]

Storytelling, and journal writing, are useful learning techniques, facilitating the discovery of practice-based knowledge.[24]

You may want to use a reflective cycle, cues or even to consider creative expression. Often we feel inadequate when it comes to creativity. However, we are limited only by our own conditioning, imagination and motivation. You may wish to:
➤ paint a picture and see what happens
➤ write a poem following a death or suicide, letting it wander until it tells you how you feel
➤ sing a song you create yourself.

Try free writing, where you just begin to write and see what happens. This can enable you to capture the richness and beauty of practice when sometimes it all feels too much. Write about incidents or practice within 24 hours to recapture the whole situation. Begin with writing down negative feelings; writing it down also helps to 'let it go'. For example, 'I feel angry because . . . or I am so sad because . . .'.[24]

Show parts of your journal to people you trust; they will help you explore deeper, and not only to challenge your attitudes and practice but to validate them. However, it takes courage to be self-critical, acknowledge our mistakes and admit that we are not always caring, and that sometimes it is difficult to cope.

SELF-ASSESSMENT EXERCISE 2.7

Time: 15 minutes
- Choose a recent incident.
- Try some form of creative expression.
- See what happens.

Learning from the individual and family

The individual and family are the biggest learning resource. Each person, if we listen, can teach us something about the experience of being ill, our assumptions and ourselves.

Furthermore, each of us has some personal experience of receiving intervention or treatment, or a family member, and/or feeling low, depressed and anxious. Maybe, even using substances to self-medicate and act as an emotional sponge. Instead of setting this to one side, and thinking of ourselves solely as professionals, reflect on this; explore what we have learnt from being on the 'receiving end'.

3 Off-job learning and development on one's own

Consider looking at other learning resources, such as:

➤ videos
➤ media
➤ Internet
➤ intranet
➤ computer-assisted learning packages
➤ e-learning programmes.

Regularly read journals, utilise books within your library and identify a particular topic or project to undertake.

SELF-ASSESSMENT EXERCISE 2.8

> **Time: 1 hour 30 minutes**
> Identify an individual or family member who you think taught you a lot.
> - What did you learn? This could be your experience as a receiver of intervention and treatment, family member or someone you have cared for.
> - With permission, interview an individual or family member about his/her experience.

CONCLUSION

One of our greatest challenges is to be ourselves. To recognise that we and we alone are the tool of effective intervention and treatment. We offer intervention and treatment for people in a society, in which mental health–substance use problems are a taboo and stigmatised. Learning to work 'as a whole' and to be truly alongside the individual in a healthcare culture, which often focuses on a narrow, clinical approach, is hard. Moreover, to have the courage to question our own and others' values, attitudes and judgements is challenging. We need to develop a lifelong approach to learning, by utilising a blended learning approach, which incorporates learning from our own experiences, practice, classroom and other learning resources. It is hoped that this chapter has helped you to consider the breadth of knowledge necessary, and ways in which you may learn. *Most important of all is your need to learn, to know, to value, and care, for yourself.*

> Actions may be positive or negative according to the intention that underlies them, just as a crystal reflects the colours of its surroundings.[25]

POST-READING EXERCISE 2.1

Time: 30 minutes
1 Identify your learning needs.
2 Develop your personal learning action plan.

Ensure you identify the most appropriate ways of learning to meet your needs.
Consider:
- Secondment?
- Mentor?
- Shadowing?
- Reflective journal?
- Team learning?
- Other?

REFERENCES

1 Page CR. *The Mirror of Existence: stepping into wholeness.* Saffron Walden: The CW Daniel Company Limited; 1995.
2 Alcohol Concern. *Fact Sheet 17: alcohol and mental health.* London: Alcohol Concern; 2004.
3 Mental Health Foundation. *Cheers? Understanding the relationship between alcohol and mental health.* London: Mental Health Foundation; 2006.
4 Mental Health Foundation. *Choosing Mental Health: a policy agenda for mental and public health.* London: Mental Health Foundation; 2005.
5 James C, Macleod R. The problematic nature of education in palliative care. *J Palliat Care.* 1993; **9**: 5–10.
6 Davies B, Oberle K. Dimensions of the supportive role of the nurse in palliative care. *Oncol Nurs Forum.* 1990; **17**: 87–94.
7 Habermas J. *Knowledge and Human Interest.* London: Heinemann; 1978.
8 Carper BA. Fundamental patterns of knowing in nursing. *Adv Nurs Sci.* 1978; **1**: 13–23.
9 Benner P. *From Novice to Expert: excellence and power in clinical practice.* Menlo Park, CA: Addison-Wesley; 1984.
10 Department of Health. *A First Class Service: quality service in the new NHS.* London: Department of Health Publications; 1998.
11 Department of Health. *The NHS Knowledge and Skills Framework (NHS KSF) and the development review process.* London: Department of Health; 2004.
12 Rogers CR. *Freedom to Learn for the 80s.* Columbus, OH: Merrill; 1983.
13 Rogers A. *Teaching Adults.* 3rd ed. Maidenhead: Open University Press; 2002.
14 Bloom BS. *Taxonomy of Educational Objectives.* London: Longman; 1965.
15 Kolb DA. *Learning Style Inventory Technical Manual.* Boston, MA: McBer; 1976.
16 Honey P, Mumford A. *Learning Style Helper's Guide.* Maidenhead: Peter Honey; 2006.
17 Sperry R, Ornstein R. In: Rose, C. *Accelerated Learning.* 4th ed. Buckingham: Accelerated Learning Publications; 1989.
18 Mok E, Man LW, Wong FK. The issue of death and dying: employing problem-based learning in nursing education. *Nurse Educ Today.* 2002; **22**: 319–29.
19 Wilkinson JM. *Nursing Process: a critical thinking approach.* Menlo Park, CA: Addison-Wesley Nursing; 1996.
20 Wilkinson S. Factors which influence how nurses communicate with cancer patients. *J Adv Nurs.* 1991; **16**: 677–88.

21 Smith P, Gray B. Reassessing the concept of emotional labour in student nurse education: role of link lecturers and mentors in a time of change. *Nurse Educ Today.* 2001; **21**: 230–7.

22 Spouse J. *Professional Learning in Nursing.* Oxford: Blackwell; 2003.

23 Gibbs G. *Learning by Doing: a guide to teaching and learning methods.* Oxford: Further Education Unit, Oxford Brooks University; 1988.

24 Johns C. *Being Mindful Easing Suffering: reflections on palliative care.* London: J Kingsley; 2004.

25 Dilgo Khyentse Pinoche. As cited in: Föllmi D, Föllmi O. *Buddhist Offerings 365 Days.* London: Thames and Hudson; 2003.

TO LEARN MORE

Barker P, editor. *Psychiatric and Mental Health Nursing: the craft of caring.* London: Arnold; 2008.

Spouse J. *Professional Learning in Nursing.* Oxford: Blackwell; 2003.

ACKNOWLEDGEMENT

© Cooper J. *Stepping into Palliative Care 1: relationships and responses.* 2nd ed. Oxford: Radcliffe Publishing; 2006. Reproduced with permission of the copyright holder.

The author is grateful to Jo Cooper, and Radcliffe Publishing Ltd, for permitting this adaptation.

CHAPTER 3

What is in a name?
The search for appropriate and consistent terminology

Phil Barker

> *Most people who bother with the matter at all would admit that the English language is in a bad way, but it is generally assumed that we cannot by conscious action do anything about it. Our civilization is decadent and our language – so the argument runs – must inevitably share in the general collapse. It follows that any struggle against the abuse of language is a sentimental archaism, like preferring candles to electric light or hansom cabs to aeroplanes.*
>
> George Orwell [1]

THE POLITICS OF LANGUAGE GAMES

The names given to different aspects of our human experience have evolved over centuries or have been developed by powerful individuals or groups for some highly specific purpose.[2] In the Western scientific tradition, the naming of 'things', through some system of *classification*, was the key to making sense of the world in which we live. It would be comforting to believe that 'names' – especially terminology – attributed to things in our world, whether within vernacular or technical vocabularies, are always neutral or 'value free'. Nowhere is this less true than in the area of jargon where a discrete professional language has been developed for a specific professional purpose. The contested term 'dual diagnosis' is but one example of a simple descriptive expression that appears to hold the power to incite heated debate.

REFLECTIVE EXERCISE 3.1

Time: 5 minutes
- What does 'dual diagnosis' mean to you?
- Make a list of the alternative terms or expressions, which you believe might mean much the same thing.

The naming of things

Whichever language we speak, its usage can prove problematic, especially when we try to express complex or contested ideas. We may *know*, implicitly, what we mean, but find it difficult to make that meaning explicit, by putting it into words. Similarly, when people hear us speak, do they always understand exactly what we *mean*, or do they *interpret* what we say? Most 'socio-political' talk is riddled with such confusion and the field of 'mental health and substance use' is no exception.

By the end of the first decade of the 21st century, 'dual diagnosis' had become firmly embedded in the health and social care language: the term of choice in many countries to refer to people with 'co-occurring mental health and alcohol and other drug issues'.[3] Although not universally popular, attempts to critique or otherwise unpack this idea might be considered vain – both pointless and self-serving. Historically, medicine led the development of services for people with such problems (or 'issues' in the contemporary parlance). Any attempt to escape the influence of 'medicalised or partisan terminology'[4] has proven difficult. Many of the problems experienced by people embraced by the 'dual diagnosis' category are interpersonal or social in nature. Since medicine provided the original framework for thinking and talking about such problems, many professionals, politicians and bureaucrats find it difficult to step beyond the medical frame of reference.

To the layperson, the idea of 'dual diagnosis' might appear straightforward: some people with 'mental health problems' also take 'illicit drugs' or alcohol. 'Substance use' is one of the oldest practices known to humankind. Alcohol and most so-called 'illicit' drugs have been used for thousands of years, in all cultures, as a means of influencing mood or other aspects of consciousness, including their use as ritualistic devices. Only recently have people involved in such 'culturally appropriate' practices been viewed as having 'mental health problems'.

It seems unremarkable, therefore, that people who experience some disturbance of their consciousness (thoughts, feelings, sense of 'self', etc.), should seek to manipulate these internal states, by 'using substances'. Effecting a change in consciousness appears to be the main reason why anyone drinks alcohol or takes drugs. The layperson is doubtless also aware that the commonest way of dealing with so-called 'mental health problems' is through the use of drugs. However, whereas drugs prescribed by a physician are considered appropriate (and legal), 'self-medicating' is invariably viewed as 'problematic' (and illegal). Ironically, I must give formal permission (consent) to a physician to give me a drug; but I must seek the physician's permission (prescription) if I wish to give myself a drug. Consequently, *any* 'substance use' by a person described as having 'mental health problems', which is not sanctioned by a 'mental health professional', becomes doubly problematic, if not further expression of the person's 'pathology'.

Two key roles of medicine have been to *name* 'disorders' or 'conditions' (taxonomy) and to *explain* their existence (pathology). Various names have been coined for different 'psychiatric' or 'substance use-related disorders', (e.g. 'schizophrenia', 'alcoholism'). However, little explanation of their 'underlying pathology' (in the strictly medical sense) has been forthcoming. At the same time, it has become commonplace to talk of the 'one in four'[5] people who are likely to experience '*mental* health problems' in their lifetime. Such statistics no longer even attempt to make any distinction between the more severe forms of 'schizophrenia' and the most minor forms of 'social anxiety'. Although carcinoma and sinusitis are both '*physical* health problems' there would likely be a public outcry if politicians and legislators conflated these two, very different conditions, in healthcare statistics. No such outrage arises in the mental health–substance use arena, perhaps because there is little agreement regarding what 'exactly' is under discussion.

Despite the absence of any discrete pathology, it is reassuring (to some) to assume that people with 'mental health problems' have some form of 'mental illness' akin to other illnesses like diabetes or anaemia. Many continue to assert a similar illness (or disease) basis for various 'addictions' or substance use problems. In cases, the 'illness' or 'disease process' serves to explain (or excuse) associated behavioural problems. Apparently, men kill their wives because they are 'insane' or 'under the influence of alcohol or drugs'. Rarely, do people appear given to uninhibited expressions of love or generosity while under similar 'influences'. In most Western societies self-control is highly valued and people are expected to take responsibility for their actions. However, where persons are given diagnoses related to 'mental illness' and/or 'drug/alcohol addiction' the expectation that they are responsible for their actions often is considerably lowered, especially in law.

REFLECTIVE EXERCISE 3.2

Time: 15 minutes
- If your family/friends thought that you were 'drinking too much', would you welcome this behaviour being 'diagnosed' as 'substance misuse' or 'addiction'? If not, why not?
- If, at the same time, you were experiencing some 'emotional' or 'psychological' problems, would you welcome 'dual diagnosis' being used to describe your situation? If not, why not?

THE NAMING OF PERSONS

Language in the health and social care fields has long had a political edge. Over the past 30 years debates have raged over the most appropriate terminology for the people who receive services for problems related to their mental health or substance use. (My preferred terms of address – *people* and *persons* – appear the least used.) The original healthcare term 'patient' is now viewed as too overtly medical, associated with its root definition implying 'suffering'. It also included an element of *passivity*, since historically patients were expected to do whatever the physician deemed necessary or appropriate.

The alternative term *client* was popularised by social workers, influenced by the work of Carl Rogers in the 1940s.[6] However, the Latin root of this term – *cliens* – referred to the subservient relationship between a *plebian* (one of the common people) and a *patrician* (aristocrat) in Roman society, who acted as a patron. Although rarely acknowledged, the term *client* also maintains the idea of a power differential between those who *offer* and those who *receive* services.[7] Some countries, like the USA and Australia, have flirted with the notion of 'consumers' in mental health and substance use services. However, few such people have anything like the free choice and rights protection available to consumers at the supermarket. In the UK, the concept of the 'service user' holds unfortunate echoes of the 'user–abuser' relationship, and in many countries the term 'user' holds unsavoury connotations (especially of exploitation or selfishness) and often is restricted solely to someone who 'uses' illicit drugs.

Like many related idioms, 'dual diagnosis' has become something of a political football. It provides a means by which a disparate range of people – lay and professional – can play the 'mental health and substance use' game. To distinguish this particular 'game' from other activities that might appear similar, special rules have been written, beginning with the naming of the 'thing', without which the game cannot be played. In a philosophical sense, 'dual diagnosis' is merely another language game.[8]

The politics of the game

Language is used in a wide variety of ways. How something is named – whether precisely or loosely – will influence how the conversation develops. At some point the key difference between the Wildlife Conservation Trust and the Cat's Protection League will be clarified by the differing nature of the 'things' in question. Over 60 years ago, George Orwell feared that the English language was in decline.

> Now, it is clear that the decline of a language must ultimately have political and economic causes: it is not due simply to the bad influence of this or that individual writer . . . [as a result language] becomes ugly and inaccurate because our thoughts are foolish, but the slovenliness of our language makes it easier to us to have foolish thoughts.[1]

One can only imagine what he might make of the bureaucratic terminology, psychobabble and examples of tortured 'newspeak' generated by political correctness – especially within health and social care,[9] which have now found their way into everyday conversation.

Linguistically, the term 'dual diagnosis' is straightforward and accurate: someone has been awarded two 'diagnoses' – one related to a 'mental health problem', the other to a 'substance use' problem. The person either complains of or exhibits two kinds of behaviour, which he/she, or others, considers 'problematic'. However, ultimately, the 'diagnosis' rests upon a set of values, regarding what is 'appropriate', 'socially acceptable' or otherwise 'normal'. The burgeoning influence of political correctness has fostered frantic attempts to develop language and terminology that is 'neutral' and avowedly 'non-judgemental' or 'inclusive'. For example, the English National Director for Mental Health offered a tortured description of 'dual diagnosis': 'mental health *illness*' associated with 'substance misuse problems'.[10] However, this also betrays the clear judgement that whereas 'substances' might be 'used' appropriately, at other times such use would be 'wrong'. The emergence of the moral panic in Western societies over the 'misuse' or 'abuse'[11] of 'substances' suggests that 'addiction' (of any kind) has become the new sin. The fashionable addition of, (e.g.) sex, shopping and Internet to the list of so-called 'addictions' suggests a growing concern to 'explain' why people cannot or will not control themselves, by reference to some imaginary 'pathology'.

Within traditional medical circles the key consideration would be – are these 'diagnoses' *valid*? Clinical or laboratory tests would confirm whether or not the patient was affected by the hypothetical condition. As noted previously, specific terminologies have been developed to name and distinguish one thing from another. Medicine developed its own terminology to help physicians be more specific and scientific about the phenomena potentially associated with illness and disease. Regrettably, in the absence of any genuine pathological basis, psychiatric diagnoses bear no relation to medical diagnosis, but merely represent linguistic, terminological agreement among psychiatrists.[12] Simply stated, dual diagnosis merely denotes that someone has been 'doubly categorised'. In principle, I could be diagnosed with any number of the hundreds of diagnostic categories within the DSM IV, not just two of them. Indeed, in some countries, like the USA, 'dual diagnosis' has been used to refer to people with an intellectual disability (mental retardation) and another psychiatric disorder.[13]

Sadly, due to the increasingly careless use of language, to which Orwell first referred, many people now talk as if 'dual diagnosis' is a *thing* in itself, rather than a social construction. For example, the Mental Health Association of New South Wales in Australia[14] talks about the large number of people '*affected* by dual diagnosis', and its 'symptoms' (emphasis added), as if this was a new condition (like 'swine flu' – at the time of writing, the latest potential pandemic).

THE POLITICS OF COMPROMISE
Problems in living

There has been much squabbling over terminology in the 'dual diagnosis' field.[4] However, although fighting with words may generate heat and smoke it may shed little light on the topic. The most popular terms – 'dual diagnosis', 'comorbidity', 'co-occurring' and 'coexisting' – suggest that the person has more than one *problem in living*. We might consider asking the following.

➤ *How* does a particular term 'work'? What does it appear to 'express'?
➤ For *whom* does it work?
➤ To what particular *purpose*?

REFLECTIVE EXERCISE 3.3

Time: 15 minutes
- Make a list of the reasons – personal, social, psychological, economic – why a service called Helping People with Problems in Living (HPPL) would be an advance on existing Dual Diagnosis Services.
- Make a list of the reasons why you think that such a HPPL service would not be possible in contemporary society.

Cooper alluded to such questions when he proposed that:

> Whatever the nature of substance use, it should be considered in the context of the individual's personal history and circumstances. Stereotypes of the substance user should be abandoned in favour of a more individualised, eclectic and holistic understanding of the person. Interventions on behalf of the person whose substance use is harmful to themselves or others should be based on thorough assessment and should involve the person.[15]

Most workers in the mental health and substance use fields would acknowledge that most of their people present with a variety of problems, rather than merely one or two. Among these are likely to be:
➤ a range of 'severe' or 'disabling' mental health problems
➤ homelessness/unstable housing
➤ increased risk of being violent
➤ increased risk of victimisation
➤ more contact with the criminal justice system
➤ family problems
➤ history of childhood abuse (sexual/physical).[16]

If professionals adopted such an 'eclectic and holistic understanding of the person', all significant problems in living might be identified and might, subsequently, be addressed given appropriate resources and commitment on the part of the person – and the professional. Indeed, focusing on addressing a person's problems in living, through some pragmatic, collaborative effort, seems little more than common sense – or perhaps it is an uncommon wisdom. Why the need for complex bureaucratic/professional jargon, like dual diagnosis or co-occurring/comorbid and so forth?

A service focused on 'problems in living' would, however, be unlikely to thrive, not because it is incorrectly named, but because it lacks the association with 'illness' or 'disability', which existing social, professional and political institutions need to justify providing it in the first place.

Szasz noted wryly that:

> When our religion was Christianity, we fasted and feasted: now that our religion is medicine, we diet and binge. Thus was gluttony replaced by obesity, prayer by psychotherapy, the monastery by the clinic, the clergyman by the clinician, the Vatican by the Food and Drug Administration, and God, for whom being slim meant being virtuous, by medicine, for which it means being healthy.[17]

Orwell believed that:

> One ought to recognize that the present political chaos is connected with the decay of language, and that one can probably bring about some improvement by starting at the verbal end. If you simplify your English, you are freed from the worst follies of orthodoxy.[1]

However, the kind of English found in contemporary mental health–substance use-services, and the socio-political influences that have shaped it, would likely bewilder even the futuristically minded Orwell. I would hope that all those involved in such services could agree on the simplest way of naming the field of practice. However, given the myriad social, philosophical, political, economic and personal influences involved, attaining such agreement – at least internationally – could take some time.

REFERENCES

1 Orwell G. Politics and the English language. In: Orwell G, *A Collection of Essays*. San Diego, CA; Harvest Books; 1946/1981. pp. 156, 158.

2 Baugh AC, Cable T. *A History of the English Language*. 4th ed. London: Routledge; 1993.

3 Staiger PK, Long C, McCabe M, *et al*. Defining dual diagnosis: a qualitative study of the views of health care workers. *Ment Health and Subst Use*. 2008; **1**: 193–204.

4 Velleman R, Baker A. Moving away from medicalised or partisan terminology: a contribution to the debate. *Ment Health Subst Use*. 2008; **1**: 2–9.

5 Kelly BD. The power gap: freedom, power and mental illness. *Soc Sci Med*. 2006; **63**: 2118–28.

6 Rogers C. Significant aspects of client-centred therapy. *Am Psychol*. 1946; **1**: 415–22.

7 Barker P, Kerr B. *The Process of Psychotherapy: the journey of discovery*. Oxford: Butterworth Heinemann; 2000. p. 4.

8 Wittgenstein L. *Philosophical Investigations*. Oxford; Blackwell; 1953/2001. p. 7.

9 Ryle A. NHS Newspeak. *Psychiatr Bull R Coll Psychiatr*. 1991; **15**: 226.

10 Department of Health. *Mental Health Policy Implementation Guide: dual diagnosis good practice guide*. London: Department of Health; 2002.

11 Emmelkamp PMG, Vedel E. *Evidence-Based Treatments for Alcohol and Drug Abuse: a practitioner's guide to theory, methods, and practice*. London: Routledge; 2006.

12 Maddux J. Stopping the 'madness': positive psychology and the deconstruction of the illness ideology and the DSM. In: CR Snyder, SJ Lopez, editors. *Handbook of Positive Psychology*. Oxford: Oxford University Press; 1996.

13 Crews W D, Bonaventura S, Rowe F. Dual diagnosis: prevalence of psychiatric disorders in a large state residential facility for individuals with mental retardation. *Am J Ment Retard*. 1994; **98**: 688–731.

14 Mental Health Association, NSW. *Dual Diagnosis*. Available at: www.mentalhealth.asn.au/images/pdf/Illness/Dual_Diagnosis.pdf (accessed 9 February 2010).

15 Cooper DB. The person who uses substances. In: P Barker, editor. *Psychiatric and Mental Health Nursing: the craft of caring*. London: Arnold; 2003.

16 Cooper P. The person who experiences mental health and substance use problems. In: P Barker, editor. *Psychiatric and Mental Health Nursing: the craft of caring*. London: Arnold; 2008.

17 Szasz TS. *Words to the Wise: a medical-philosophical dictionary*. New Brunswick, NJ: Transaction Publishers; 2004. p. 98.

CHAPTER 4

The mental health–substance use journey

Caroline O'Grady

INTRODUCTION

The journey through mental health–substance use problems is a long, arduous road. Individuals who experience ill health almost always 'live it' for many years, even decades. That person's life can be interrupted by periods of active symptoms, highlighted by periods of remission and recovery. Each illness has symptoms that hinder the person's ability to function effectively and cope interpersonally. Not only is the individual affected by two or more separate illnesses, but the mental health–substance use problems interact with one another – exacerbate each other – predisposing the person to relapses. At times symptoms can overlap, mask or mimic each other, making diagnosis, intervention and treatment perplexing. In addition, there is no single type mental health–substance use problem. Consequently, a variety of different forms of mental health–substance use problems are possible. They are commonly accompanied by:

➤ family problems
➤ interpersonal difficulties
➤ isolation
➤ social withdrawal
➤ financial problems
➤ employment problems
➤ school problems
➤ high risk behaviours
➤ legal problems
➤ multiple healthcare issues
➤ increased emergency room admissions
➤ multiple admissions to intervention and treatment services
➤ homelessness.

Ongoing difficulties with recovery over time may trigger feelings of failure and alienation. However, perhaps the greatest tragedy is the damage that occurs to individuals due to stigma, prejudice and discrimination.

People with mental health–substance use problems struggle, not only with the symptoms and the many disabling ramifications of the disorders, but are challenged by the prejudice and discrimination that so often accompanies conditions that are commonly misunderstood, feared, avoided and rejected. People who experience mental health–substance use problems, and their families, frequently note that the associated stigma can be far worse than the actual illnesses.[1] Stigma can become a powerful taint on one's identity and take a terrible toll on a person's overall quality of life. Many individuals struggle with a double burden:

➤ the debilitating effects of the illness
➤ the equally debilitating effects of stigmatisation.

REFLECTIVE PRACTICE EXERCISE 4.1

Time: 15 minutes
● What does the word 'stigma' mean to you?
● Consider how this might impact on the individual and family.

What might the consequences of stigma be during the life journey for the individual and family?

Stigma is a powerful social phenomenon that dramatically alters the way people view themselves and are viewed as persons. An early report defined stigma as

> a series of myths which serves only to quarantine the mentally ill [and addicted] from the rest of society. It brands the person seeking professional services with a mark of shame . . . stigma isolates and punishes those in need of help. It creates for individuals with mental health a sense of impotency against achieving normalcy, of being acceptable within society.[2]

One author noted that stigma has retained much of its original connotations – people continue to use differences to exile or avoid others.[3] The complexity of a problem like stigma is enormous and has implications for us all:

➤ personal
➤ societal
➤ family
➤ community
➤ socio-economic
➤ health-related.

In addition to the social effects, stigma can have negative and long-lasting consequences on self-esteem. When it comes to ill health problems, such as mental illness–substance use, the etiological factors, and the consequences of stigma, prejudice and discrimination are profound, historically based, and are not, nor will they continue to be, easily reduced or eradicated.

KATE'S STORY

Throughout this chapter Kate's story will use – or rather, this brief narrative will serve to skim the surface of – a more than 30-year journey of suffering and recovery from mental health–substance use problems. The objective of this chapter is to give the reader a glimpse into Kate's journey, using her own words. Kate has given permission to relay this story here in the hope that it might bring about change. To do justice to Kate's narrative an attempt will be made to emphasise how stigma, prejudice and discrimination impacted heavily on each stage of her journey and how the professional can make a difference, both in fighting stigma, and advocating for the individual and family; or in actually perpetuating, even exacerbating, the destructive impact of stigma.

Beginning the journey

Kate: Being the middle of three daughters, I was kept very sheltered by two older parents who could best be described as highly overprotective, fearful and fairly controlling but loving and very giving. I could never really accept that the day would come when I would not be with them any more. I needed them for everything – I was afraid to do anything on my own. I cried easily as a child and was very reactive to anything upsetting, but beyond years of bedwetting (for which I was very ashamed – it was kept a family secret for 12 years), I didn't think too much about feeling a bit different from other kids. It would be an understatement to describe myself as overly attached to my parents and thus it was not surprising that after I moved 50 miles away to university at the age of 19, I barely managed to maintain a sense of stability and my usual excellent academic record. I continued to achieve high grades in my first year of university for seven months before succumbing to symptoms of depression and anxiety. At that point, I could no longer stop crying and pacing alone in my dorm room. Every weekend I made frantic trips home and I was greatly reluctant to return to the university. Eventually, I stopped going to my classes in other parts of the campus and I completely isolated myself in my dorm room. This isolation eventually developed into an obsession with weight control, incessant exercise, a refusal to eat and a preoccupation with body image that led to a significant weight loss of 30 pounds from my already slim frame. An admission to the local hospital emergency room and then to a medical unit for starvation eventually led to an assessment by a mental health team and an involuntary transfer to the psychiatry department. Up to that point, I had been hiding my sadness and pain as best I could, but I was living 24 hours a day in fear of disclosure; I felt so ashamed of myself, I was worried about disappointing and hurting my parents, afraid of being called 'crazy' and convinced that since I had been 'committed' to a mental health inpatient unit, my opportunities in life had ended. Up to that point, I had still managed to 'save face' and hide how much I was suffering, but worrying about being found out caused so much anxiety and preoccupation – but now it was all out in the open and everyone would know and laugh or would no longer want anything to do with me. I did not stop to think about where these ideas were coming from – all I knew was that many of them were reinforced by the attitudes and behaviour of many of the people I had known my whole life and, eventually, by many health professionals. My shame and embarrassment were overwhelming and I felt like all possible opportunities had been squashed because of my own weakness.

Kate had begun to experience the early impact of her illness and of having a mental health diagnosis. In her mind, the psychiatric hospitalisation meant that she was now 'discredited' – all hopes and dreams of a professional career in medicine or nursing were lost. Certain attributes, such as particular psychiatric disorders, and drug and alcohol problems, become heavily stigmatised, especially when their discrediting effects are deep and very extensive.[3] It questions whether a stigmatised person assumes his/her differentness is already known about by the public (in which case, the stigmatised person is deemed *discredited*), or whether it is neither known nor perceivable by others (the person is still safe but is *discreditable*, or in danger of being 'discovered').[3] Kate not only had the burden of her ill health – she was also feeling the burden of external and internal stigma, and had moved from the stress, preoccupation and worry that her problems might be discovered, to fear about how she would be treated by others now that her problems had been exposed.

REFLECTIVE PRACTICE EXERCISE 4.2

Time: 20 minutes
As you read on, consider the knowledge, skills and attitude of the professional involved in Kate's admission.
- How does empirical knowledge and aesthetic/intuitive knowledge impact on Kate as an individual?
- Make a list of the 'helping' conditions you noticed.

*Kate: After I was moved to the psychiatric ward that first time, I was so scared that I wouldn't leave my hospital room or talk to co-patients or to any professionals . . . except for one family doctor whom I had met on the medical unit and who continued to come over to see me (and did so for the entire six months of that initial mental health admission). I have to say that there was something about her – she was really professional, but really knowledgeable – and caring at the same time. She was one busy lady – but she always took that extra 15 minutes to sit by my bed and talk with me. She looked me straight in the eye and it made me feel important, like my feelings actually mattered to somebody. I looked forward to her visits every day – and I listened closely to what she had to say because she listened to me. She told me that she didn't think of people who had problems like mine as 'crazy' – she thought of sick people as being in a state of 'dis-ease' or as experiencing a 'lack of ease'. She helped me move past my emotional paralysis, shame and fear and because of her, I was eventually able to open up and develop a strong working relationship with a few of the nurses and the resident psychiatrist. I had never been able to talk before, never in my life had I talked about how I felt or what I thought. You just didn't do that in my family. You were **told** what you thought, and you simply didn't talk about how you felt. That's why this experience was so different for me. To this day, over 30 years later, I still think about that doctor and what she did for me. I'll never forget her. The nurses took what I had to say seriously, but they had a pretty quick sense of humour too. My high school teachers used to say that I had an edge, a cynical view of the world and a sharp sense of humour. I enjoyed laughing and it was one of the few things that could naturally ease my nervousness – as long as others took me seriously when the situation required. Those nurses were gifted – or maybe they were just being themselves, being human beings – I felt like one of them sometimes, a part of a group. They used to tell me funny stories from their own lives,* *jokes (sometimes about the doctors), and occasionally helped me to see the humorous side of situations about which I could only feel anger and injustice. That really took a lot of skill and a good sense of timing! They even went out of their way to bring a guest in to visit with me – this person had previously been an inpatient on the same unit and had been discharged a year earlier. She was currently back in school full-time and had returned to her old hobbies of drawing and singing. She really gave me a lot of hope. Altogether, the staff made me feel like I had a say in my own life, that my opinions and feelings were valued, that I was an intelligent, worthwhile person with a pretty quick sense of humour and that I had what it took to become anything I wanted to in life. I was 20 years old and they had given me a glimmer of hope.*

The professionals involved in Kate's first inpatient admission made a very significant and positive difference not only in her own self-esteem and self-confidence, and in the remission of her presenting problems, but in her sense of hopefulness and value as a human being. Their therapeutic skills and knowledge went a long way towards helping Kate with both her mental health symptoms and with the pain she was enduring due to stigma.

These professionals demonstrated great respect for Kate as a person and as an intelligent, unique individual with decision-making capacity and autonomy. They treated Kate as another human being rather than as a diagnosis, and avoided making assumptions and quick judgements about her behaviours, choosing instead to interpret them as the non-verbal expressions of someone who had never had the opportunity to learn how to articulate her thoughts and feelings, or learn how to validate and take care of herself. They also normalised her illness by talking about how common depression and anxiety were among the general population and about the high prevalence of eating disorders in young women attending university. Instead of using terms like 'pathology' and 'disorder', they explained that the word 'dis-ease' could easily be thought of as a universal human condition – a state of suffering, a lack of ease or calm; and they explained that her symptoms and behaviours were indicative of deeper longstanding struggles. Moreover, the professionals encouraged Kate to complete her first-year course exams while she was an inpatient. In essence, the professionals were human beings that treated Kate like a human being – even shared their own personal stories about illnesses, and traits for which they had been stigmatised, and how this had impacted upon them. They offered, and were open to sharing, education and information about Kate's particular problems. Moreover, the professionals gave Kate an opportunity to meet a woman recovering from the same illness – a person who was leading a successful and fulfilling life after struggling for years with similar problems. This was a remarkably hope-inspiring strategy for a young person frightened that her life was over and all hope and dreams crushed because of a psychiatric label.

One of the most important factors – one that had a hugely significant and positive effect on Kate – involved a 'skill' that as professionals we know is essential, but that we sometimes take for granted. It can be summed up in a single word – *listening*. We all know the importance of assessing the symptoms, and of assessing a person's motivation to make changes and readiness-to-change. Hopefully, we realise the significance of asking the family questions, becoming family-responsive – but do we really know how to *listen*? Are we able to sit still and do this? We know how to ask questions – and we hear and record the person's responses in detail, and ensure that these are documented accurately – but are we able to sit and truly *listen* to that person? To 'not talk' but, rather, to 'be with', facilitating that person to tell his/her story – the way it is in that particular moment.

Further along the journey: moving into deep suffering

Kate: *During this first of what ended up to be over 50 hospitalisations (including inpatient stays, crisis admissions, emergency room visits, short- and long-term stays in various substance use treatment centres, etc.) over the course of a 25-year period, I met Leah, another patient who became a very good friend of mine. In one sense, it was great that I developed a friendship with someone who shared a similar diagnosis – we had many laughs and long talks and we were able to help each other through many difficult times; but in another sense, such a friendship had a destructive element to it. Leah mentioned that she had discovered a way to help suppress her appetite and control her anxiety at the same time and she did this by using double or triple the recommended dose of anti-nausea medication and antihistamines (the latter is a medication taken for allergy symptoms). She said they were harmless, you could buy them on the shelf in any drug store and they were very inexpensive. In fact, Leah was kind enough to pick some up for me on one of her overnight passes from the hospital. She recommended that I do the same as her – to get the appetite suppressant effect, take two to three times the recommended dose of both medications – they would also help me to sleep, she said. In my rapidly changing state of anxious desperation and depression at that time, it struck me that if two to three times the recommended dose worked so well, then 10 times the recommended dose would work even better! Let me just say that this overdose did indeed suppress my appetite – it also caused nausea and vomiting and worsened my anxiety and depression to such a level that I was on the brink of suicide. But before the more unpleasant side-effects struck, these little pills also helped me forget about all of my problems for a few hours. And that's all I thought about afterwards. That initial experience of abusing seemingly harmless, everyday, easily accessible, legal, commonly used medication led me to do it again the very next time I was feeling extremely depressed and nervous, which happened as soon as the side-effects from the initial overdose had worn off. Suddenly, my entire recovery was thrown off course. I didn't know what was going on – I was getting so much worse and I was more and more confused and depressed. Eventually, overuse of these pills would make my mental health symptoms so unbearable that I would be literally unable to function. But all that mattered in the moment was how unbearably sad and nervous and guilty and scared I felt and how I couldn't stand feeling that way any more – and that taking a handful of these pills helped me to forget my problems and my emotions for maybe four hours, even if recovering from the side-effects of such an overdose could take as much as four to five days and lead to weeks of suffering from an exacerbation of all the rest of my psychiatric symptoms. That initial one incident of overuse of these so-called harmless drugs would lead to 20 years of extreme daily abuse of this medication that in the end only served to intensify my depression, anxiety, rage, emotional dysregulation, worsen my inability to work or study consistently or live independently; and it resulted in frantic self-destructive behaviours such as the cutting of my arms, legs and throat.*

Looking back now, I think if I had been a 'good' patient, simply said 'thank you' at the end of my first six-month hospitalisation and gone back home to continue my life after

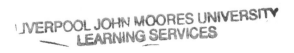

discharge, everything might have turned out differently. But I now understand that this just doesn't happen very often when people have many overlapping problems, some of them psychiatric in nature and some related to abuse of alcohol and/or other drugs. I used to think I was 'different', 'weird', even within the mental health system because I had so many problems, I couldn't seem to get over them and I couldn't seem to get better – I was 'complicated'. Once again, I started feeling like I had done something wrong, that I was weak, I should be ashamed of myself, I should work harder to figure out what was wrong with me and do something to rectify the situation – after all, wasn't I supposed to be an intelligent person? Did my constant failing mean that I was actually stupid and had been fooling myself all this time? Or was I really just lazy? Of course, I now realise that co-occurring mental illness and substance use problems do not just go away simply because we decide we are going to work harder on them or ignore them. But for many, many years, and I am only scratching the surface of my journey here, I couldn't figure out why I wasn't able to (and it was suggested at one point that I chose not to) get better. That first hospitalisation was only the beginning of a 30-year long journey, three-quarters of which I suffered anxiety, depression, extreme anger, hopelessness, grief and loss, abandonment and self-destructiveness. My journey through this illness, I am still embarrassed to admit, consisted of over 50 hospitalisations, several of these greater than four to six months in length, in addition to several crisis and emergency admissions, short and long-term stays at addiction treatment centres in two countries, several attempts at self-help/mutual aid support groups and treatment from over 30 psychiatrists and an impossible-to-count number of nurses and other healthcare professionals. I have been given so many diagnoses (I'm not sure I can remember them all) from various healthcare professionals over these many years including Major Depression, Generalized Anxiety Disorder, Separation Anxiety, Attachment Disorder, Substance Abuse Disorder, Substance Dependence Disorder, Bipolar Disorder, Borderline Personality Disorder, Anorexia Nervosa, Bulimia Nervosa, Dependent Personality Disorder – and finally, complex Post-traumatic Stress Disorder. I had so many labels; I didn't even know who I was any more.

Kate's discussion of the sheer number and variety of diagnoses, given over the years by different professionals, brings to mind a comment made by Patricia Deegan, a disability-rights advocate, psychologist and researcher.[4] Most important, Deegan herself is a psychiatric survivor and activist, psychologist and consultant to government and community-based mental health agencies, and a known advocate of the mental health recovery movement.[4] She has spoken around the world about her personal and professional experience of recovery. In particular, she has described the restriction in freedom of expression and choice experienced by many people who have suffered from mental health problems and refers to the forcing of diagnostic labels upon people as a 'type of violence'. After her own many experiences of being referred to as a 'schizophrenic', she describes her feelings in the following way:

> [I felt] the violence of being dehumanised and having my individuality reduced to a generic diagnosis. I am describing the arrogant and unapologetically clinical gaze that captures me, re-interprets me and hands me back to myself as damaged goods; disabled ... 'not-right'; broken-brained ... genetically

defective; a 'special' person with 'special' needs requiring special services in segregated places.[4]

These comments underline how crucial it is that we, the 'professionals', be extra vigilant about how we talk to the individual and the family. We need to be cautious about the language we use to describe people, and about the ways in which 'diagnostic terms' can all too easily obliterate personhood. In this way, Patricia Deegan became 'a schizophrenic'; Kate initially became 'an anorexic' and finally 'a traumatised depressed borderline substance abuser'.

External and internal stigma

Kate: *In spite of slow steps forward (that were interrupted by a lot of relapses!), throughout these many dark years, I have also been given many, shall we say, less formal diagnoses and descriptions by mental health professionals – these included 'lazy', 'chronic', 'hopeless', 'ungrateful', 'attention-seeking', 'annoying', 'crazy', 'manipulative' and 'selfish'. I was told I should feel badly for using healthcare dollars (when they should have been used for people who were really sick), I was 'stupid' (for my inability to use the help offered to me), and 'childish' (for taking up precious hospital space with my frivolous behavioural tantrums when people with 'real sickness and injuries' needed the beds). In fact, one doctor said to me, 'You're not even interested in getting better'; and a nurse on night shift during one of my longer inpatient admissions introduced herself and then added, '. . . and by the way, don't start anything tonight, I don't put up with nonsense from girls like you – I'll call security faster than you can blink, my dear'. A few years later, after a particularly desperate and depressed period in my life, I made a rather serious suicide attempt by overdosing on Tylenol. An emergency room nurse in a large teaching hospital angrily grabbed a nasogastric tube for administration of charcoal [a common emergency treatment intervention for ingestion of certain toxic chemicals] and jammed it down into my stomach. I could feel the tube gouging into the inside of my abdomen and it started causing severe pain – I knew that something was wrong (this wasn't the first time I had experienced this intervention) and when my complaints were ignored, I was forced to pull out the tube. My intention was not to be 'non-compliant' – I just couldn't stand the stabbing pain in my stomach anymore. The staff, however, became enraged and pulled me off the emergency room bed, threw my clothes over to me and said, 'Just go home – we don't help people who don't want any help. You're wasting our time'. I went home feeling that I had been punished and humiliated by the emergency room staff. Yet, at the same time, a part of me felt that they were justified in their actions and I again questioned whether I did, in fact, deserve to be medically (not to mention respectfully) treated for something that I myself had caused. This blending of anger, hurt, shame and self-hatred led to further feelings of confusion and depression. Yet another time, after I had taken an overdose on a closed ward observation unit, an exasperated nurse cursed and whispered to a colleague that I 'was the worst borderline they have ever had on that unit – and why were they even admitting me any more?' Although I didn't open my eyes, I heard the entire conversation and I will never forget it. These experiences happened over and over again for so many years, I stopped counting and eventually started thinking about no longer trying. I just kept on failing over and over again and other people kept hating me more and more – there was nowhere to go.*

These examples represent only a few from hundreds related by Kate as she narrates her journey through the horrors of mental illness and substance use in an oftentimes intolerant, ignorant, even abusive healthcare system. Discrimination is not specific to the mental health–substance use services. People with mental health–substance use problems experience discrimination in the general healthcare system – views are often dismissed and ignored, treated disrespectfully in emergency rooms and in primary care. In addition, concerns about admitting to having mental illness or substance use problems are legitimate since physical concerns may be attributed to psychological stress, anxiety or drug use and then disregarded, minimised or invalidated.

Mental health–substance use problems are enduring in nature. Although some may be resolved in a matter of months, more (chronic) problems, such as severe mental illness, personality disorders, refractory depression and bipolar disorder and substance use problems can continue, or wax and wane for many years, even decades. For many people, recovery is a lifelong journey. Relapses in mental health and substance use are common. Oftentimes, a person will experience symptoms for years, and the symptoms themselves will change over time. For Kate, although the more intensive period of her initial presenting problem (eating disorder) occurred before, and during, the first few years of her involvement in the healthcare system, other symptoms soon developed and evolved to become even greater priorities due to the nature of the risk element involved. The use of substances grew to occasionally include alcohol bingeing, the extreme use of antihistamines and anti-nausea medication and led to use of anti-anxiety medications, and repeated hospitalisations, for fall-related head injuries, and other accidents. These problems themselves were more than enough for any human being to suffer, and yet she endured the painful effects of both external and internal stigma as well.

Kate: I think the absolute worst point for me came when I realised that every door was being closed in my face. Every single person was tired of me or angry with me – there wasn't one healthcare professional that could even look at me without derision or speak to me without a cutting, angry, sarcastic edge. Everybody was fed up with me. I was upset with them, thinking, 'I didn't do this on purpose – I didn't want or ask for any of this – I wanted to be like everybody else' . . . but I also felt responsible and ashamed. At the same time, I was still desperate with no one to talk to and nowhere to go. But the message I kept getting . . . was that I had used up all of my collateral, and then some – and that the best thing for everyone would be for me to just go away and not come back.

REFLECTIVE PRACTICE EXERCISE 4.3

Time: 15 minutes
As you read through Kate's story, notice your own feelings.
- How is this making you feel?
- Do any of your feelings mirror those of Kate?
- Are there any differences?
- Do any of your feelings, even mildly, mirror those of the professionals involved?

Be honest with your responses!

After many years of similar experiences, Kate began feeling that there was nothing she could do or say that would convince people she was the same person that she had always been, with the same intelligence, sense of humour, love of animals and interest in the workings of the human mind. She realised that after many years of being moved to a locked psychiatric unit in various hospitals for repeated self-harm attempts, where she was followed around like a criminal 24 hours a day, and after one stigmatising and humiliating episode after another, she would either have to find a way to keep this part of her life a secret, or try to cope with the consequences of being other-than-human, 'not-quite-normal'. She decided that the best way to do this was to self-isolate.

Why do we stigmatise the kinds of illnesses that Kate experienced? Is it because we do not perceive them as illnesses, but instead as volitional behavioural problems from characterologically flawed individuals? There are many reasons why even mental health–substance use professionals might be prone to stigmatising certain forms of mental ill health and substance use, including stigma based on fear of violence, and stigma due to hopelessness. But stigma often accompanies disorders for which people are considered responsible and these are frequently, but not always, conditions of the mind rather than the body. It is disturbing how a particular health state becomes 'deviant' and how in cases of certain illnesses (such as depressive disorders, anxiety, borderline personality disorder and harmful substance use), there is a moralistic judgement of blame, with the individual and the family being held responsible for the ill health.[5] This tendency to blame the individual or the family remains evident today. In fact, professionals have withheld respect and care from certain people whose problems have resulted from substance use, 'character (personality) disorders' and suicidal behaviour. Such ill health may be stigmatised to the extent that they are attributed to personal culpability on the part of the individual and the family. According to this theory of 'attribution of responsibility', beliefs about personal responsibility for ill health determine negative emotional reactions, such as:

➤ rejection
➤ hostility
➤ avoidance
➤ prejudicial beliefs.

It seems that certain people are less deserving of care because they are perceived to have made a choice and brought the problems on themselves! Such conditions tend to be those least likely to arouse professional compassion and empathy.

Ultimately, Kate spoke at length about another 'incredibly compassionate, caring, direct, empowering and unique' professional – a physician specialising in the treatment of substance use problems – who would be key in helping her to turn her life around. Kate recalled that the professional never gave up on her – that eye contact was always maintained, and although the professional was caring and concerned, the expectation that Kate take charge of her own life and to direct her own recovery was clear. This professional had that special ability to *listen*, or perhaps just treated other people as he himself expected to be treated – like a valued human being.

As professionals, we can learn a number of important lessons from Kate's story. In addition to being able to sit with, and *listen* to, people that come to us, the 'professional', for help, it is important to see the individual and the family as 'guests'.[6] In this sense, we become 'hosts'.[6] According to this model of care, professionals (hosts) have an ethical, and moral, obligation to welcome the individual (guests) openly and warmly, without judgement, prejudice or exclusion.[6] This welcoming approach, in a spirit of kindness and generosity, is just as important as the ability to work effectively and competently with people based on best practice evidence.

We tend to see people at the peaks in their ill health – during crises and emergencies, during times of relapse, especially if we are working on inpatient units. Unless we are following people for years and even decades, we may not see people when they are well – because they do not come back during these periods of life stability. Seeing people constantly leaving and returning may leave some professionals feeling cautious and pessimistic, with little hope of recovery. Sometimes we may develop a sense of hopelessness and helplessness and this too can contribute to stigma. In spite of these feelings, we play an important role in 'holding the hope' for the individual and the family during the times when they are unable to do so themselves. Holding the hope means continuing to believe in people no matter how bleak the situation seems to them and in spite of any discussions about 'chronicity and treatment failures'.

REFLECTIVE PRACTICE EXERCISE 4.4

Time: 20 minutes
Consider, in some depth, the concept of 'hope'.
- How could you, as a professional, encourage hopefulness in a person who is feeling both hopeless and helpless?
- How might 'respectfulness' and 'valuing' encourage hope?

We must realise that stigma comes in many forms. Sometimes we can be well-meaning in our intentions and in an effort to shield the individual from an overabundance of stress, and a resultant relapse, due to 'vulnerability'. We may be reluctant to encourage the individual to pursue his/her interests and dreams, or we may end up speaking in a patronising manner. Consequently, the individual feels like a child, and is excluded from decisions about his/her life. As professionals, we need to ask ourselves, are we making assumptions about this individual's capacity to be responsible? Do we fear that he/she will suffer a setback due to 'vulnerability'? Everyone deserves to be given sufficient information about their ill health, and about the interventions and treatment options. Whenever possible, these discussions must take place without the overt or covert threat of coercive treatment.[7] It is vital that we reframe the relationships with the individual and family within a more *empowering partnership model*, in which we readily share education, up-to-date information and resources. Professional practice, based on such an empowerment-based model, is incongruent with talking 'at' the individual and the family, as if each does not have a mind – a choice; this is patronising and condescending.

It is important that we try to *help people deal with and overcome the disabling effects of self-stigmatisation*, or internalised stigma. This phenomenon occurs when an individual comes to share the same beliefs as others and view themselves in similarly disparaging ways. Self-stigma is:

the enemy within – it renders a person complicit with the injustice of externally imposed discrimination and stereotyping. People come to expect that they deserve to be treated poorly and to be devalued, disrespected and ignored or ostracised.[7]

Kate's narrative illustrated how deeply her own fears about having her illness disclosed and exploited affected her for so many years. We must remain cognisant that internalised stigma does not suddenly arise out of the blue. Some stigma is so historically and societally embedded that we receive messages throughout our lives underlining and even encouraging the avoidance and exclusion of certain groups of people. However, a great deal of internalised stigma is based on actual externally based stigmatising experiences, including those sometimes inflicted by health professionals.

A recovery-based philosophy and programme may serve as a partial solution to the agony of self-stigma – people become empowered, and learn to develop new coping mechanisms and skills, such as achieving increased self-awareness and self-confidence. The individual is able to cognitively reframe situations that permit that individual to let go of the negative opinions and behaviours of stigmatising others, choose to be with positive, accepting and understanding people, and move forward with what is truly important in his/her life. For many people in recovery, self-help/mutual aid support groups can greatly assist with feelings of belonging and acceptance, and simultaneously offer new ways to cope with ill health, stigma and discrimination.

As professionals, and individuals ourselves, we can also *become culturally competent* and sensitive. Many cultures hold hugely stigmatising and discriminatory attitudes towards mental health–substance use, and have set ideas about the aetiological factors underlying ill health. The individual may come to the professional bearing the burden of deep shame and embarrassment, and may hold strong beliefs about the origins and causes of his/her symptoms. The professional must be sensitive to these beliefs. This person may have experienced stigma due to any number of factors based on race, religion, skin colour, new immigration status, language and so on. The professional must be aware of the additive effects of multiple layers of stigma. It is wise to keep in mind that any human trait can be ostracised depending on the era and culture in which we happen to be born and live. Any one of us can be stigmatised for any variety of traits simply because of where we are, and at what point in time we find ourselves.

The professional should *expect complexity* rather than be surprised and annoyed by the individual who presents with complex problems and situations. Live by the motto 'complexity is the norm, not the exception'. Human beings are complex creatures and mental health–substance use problems are complex. As professionals, we must be prepared for this in terms of:

➤ education
➤ research
➤ clinical competence.

We have to be ready to offer information and education about mental health–substance use problems. If we do not have all of the answers, we must be able to refer the individual or the family to the appropriate person, service or resource. In addition, we must work on enhancing the integration of mental health–substance use intervention and treatment systems, beginning with improved communication, and sharing of information and knowledge. It is being discriminated against for having complex problems for the individual to be discharged because of a drug problem, only to be told: *'We cannot help you until you stop using drugs – you'll just have to get that problem dealt with and come back and maybe then you will be ready to work on your mood disorder'*. Conversely, for the individual to be refused acceptance into an intervention and treatment programme due to active symptoms of mental ill health that requires psychotropic medications is also discriminatory. The problem here does not lie with the individual or the family – the responsibility lies with the professional and the healthcare system. We have to develop the knowledge, skill and ability to work at even the most basic level with people who walk into our lives. Increasingly, it is the rule rather than the exception that the individual comes forward with a mental health and substance use problem. At the very least, we can:

➤ have a kind and welcoming attitude
➤ listen
➤ ask the right questions
➤ offer the most up-to-date information and education
➤ facilitate movement in the right direction.

Perhaps most importantly, a top priority for each professional who willingly chooses to specialise in these areas is to *'look within ourselves'* and reflect upon what we find there. This may very well be the most difficult strategy because it requires genuine honesty and an intimate conversation with oneself. It requires that we open our eyes to our own demons, and to think about how we might be adding to the suffering of another individual through the process of stigmatisation. Do we tend to be more intolerant of persons with certain types of problems? Do we know why this is so? Does this happen more when we are overworked and stressed (which, sadly, has become commonplace for many of us these days); if so, what can we do to ensure that we are taking care of ourselves? If we do not attend to our own emotional and physical health, the ramifications will affect more than ourselves – they will increasingly manifest as anger, hostility and exclusion towards each other, and, most importantly, towards the individual and the family who enter our lives. This is unacceptable. We need to work within one simple policy – *zero tolerance for intolerance*. We cannot change hundreds of years of stigma and discrimination towards the individual experiencing mental health–substance use problems – and we cannot change the world by ourselves. However, we can each model a spirit of kindness, compassion and tolerance for every individual who we meet in our professional and personal life. We can try to work and live by the adage: *'Let it begin with me'*.[8]

REFERENCES

1 The Public Health Agency of Canada. *A Report on Mental Illnesses in Canada*. Available at: www.phac-aspc.gc.ca/publicat/miic-mmac/pdf/men_ill_e.pdf (accessed 8 March 2010).
2 Clausen JA. Stigma and mental disorder: phenomena and terminology. *Psychiatry*. 1981; **44**: 287–96.

3 Goffman E. *Stigma: notes on the management of spoiled identity.* Englewood Cliffs, NJ: Prentice-Hall; 1963.

4 Deegan PE. Rethinking Rehabilitation: freedom. *Proceedings of the 20th World Congress of Rehabilitation International: Rethinking Rehabilitation.* 22 June 2004. Available at: www.centerforself-determination.com/docs/mh/rethinkingRehab1.pdf (accessed 8 March 2010).

5 Friedson E. Disability as deviance. In: Sussman MB, editor. *Sociology and Rehabilitation.* Washington, DC: American Sociological Association; 1965. pp. 71–99.

6 Frank AW. *The Renewal of Generosity: illness, medicine and how to live.* Chicago, IL: University of Chicago Press; 2004.

7 Mood Disorders Society of Canada. *Stigma: the hidden killer.* Available at: www.mooddisorders canada.ca/documents/Publications/Stigma%20the%20hidden%20killer.pdf (accessed 8 March 2010).

8 Miller S, Jackson J. *Let There be Peace on Earth.* Available at: www.quotegarden.com/peace.html (accessed 8 March 2010).

TO LEARN MORE

Arboledo-Florez J, Sartorius N. *Understanding the Stigma of Mental Illness: theory and interventions.* Chichester: John Wiley and Sons; 2008.

Corrigan PW. *On the Stigma of Mental Illness: practical strategies for research and social change.* Washington, DC: American Psychological Association; 2005.

Corrigan PW, Lundin R. *Don't Call Me Nuts: coping with the stigma of mental illness.* Tinley Park, IL: Recovery Press; 2001.

Hinshaw SP. *The Mark of Shame: stigma of mental illness and an agenda for change.* New York, NY: Oxford University Press; 2007.

Skinner WJ, editor. *Treating Concurrent Disorders: a guide for counsellors.* Toronto, ON: Centre for Addiction and Mental Health; 2005.

ACKNOWLEDGEMENT
Kate, thank you. May this contribute to bringing change!

A matter of human rights: people's right to healthcare for mental health–substance use

Charlotte de Crespigny, Peter Athanasos,
Jacky Talmet, Anne Wilson and Janice Elliott

PRE-READING EXERCISE 5.1

Time: 20 minutes
An individual is offered substandard, or no, healthcare because of his/her race or presenting health problem(s).
- How could this situation impact on this individual?
- How would you advocate for him/her?
- What might stop you from advocating for him/her?
- What would enable you to advocate for him/her?

INTRODUCTION
The World Health Organization (WHO) defines health in their constitution as a:

> state of complete physical, mental and social well-being and not merely the absence of disease or infirmity. The enjoyment of the highest attainable standard of health is one of the fundamental rights of every human being without distinction of race, religion, political belief, economic or social condition.[1]

This chapter provides an overview of issues related to people's right to healthcare for mental health–substance use and related physical problems. From an Australian perspective we describe various situations where people's right to healthcare was denied, and some solutions formulated.

We know that many professionals make a real difference to how people with mental health–substance use problems are treated 'on the ground'. These professionals are well trained, supported by their organisations and, importantly, are comfortable in communicating with these individuals.

KEY POINT 5.1

Respect and non-judgemental attitudes are pivotal to positive engagement and outcomes.

Despite this, at the 'ground level', people who present with mental health–substance use problems regularly receive no care, or substandard care. This occurs in general hospitals, primary health settings, mental health services, specialist substance use services, and in the juvenile justice system.[2,3] A predetermining factor is the stereotyped and judgemental attitudes of health professionals and organisation leaders.[4–8]

Health professionals can make a difference. We present information, gathered from the literature and reports by drug and alcohol nurses, to demonstrate this. While we discuss the issue from an Australian perspective, we hope that it will inform the professional in a range of settings. 'Real life' case scenarios are presented. Discussion and key questions enable readers to reflect on, and formulate, approaches in their own context.

HEALTHCARE: A BASIC HUMAN RIGHT

In 2008, Ban Ki-moon, Secretary-General of the World Health Organization, declared: *'No one should be stigmatised or discriminated against because of their dependence on drugs'.*[9] This is underscored in the Charter for People's Health Preamble, which states:

> Health is a social, economic and political issue and above all a fundamental human right. Inequality, poverty, exploitation, violence and injustice are at the root of ill health and the deaths of poor and marginalised people.[10]

The People's Health Movement Charter (p. 10) *'calls on people of the world to . . . pressure governments to adopt, implement and enforce national health and drugs policies'.*[10] Australia, New Zealand, Canada and the United Kingdom have drug policies that recognise that substance use problems are health problems. Despite this, at times, people with mental health–substance use problems continue to receive poor care, or no care at all.

THE EVIDENCE

The literature was comprised of:
➤ refereed articles
➤ Australian national policies
➤ coronial and police report[11]
➤ critical incident hospital reports
➤ anecdotal information from substance use professionals.[12]

Many reports indicate that refusal to provide safe healthcare has directly resulted in a range of negative outcomes. These include:
➤ further emotional distress
➤ exacerbation of mental health–substance use conditions

➤ untreated injuries and illnesses
➤ the final consequence, in some cases, has been avoidable disability, or death.

FACTORS
It is known that when people with mental health–substance use concerns and dilemmas present to emergency departments (ED), they risk being inappropriately assessed, as being 'just drunk' or seeking attention. This is despite the critical responsibility that the professional has in providing non-judgemental healthcare to all those in need.[13–15]

Strong and compassionate leadership can build a positive culture within care delivery teams. Unfortunately, the evidence suggests that the culture in many care delivery teams is not always positive. The acute presentations that are misdiagnosed are many. Coronial and police reports describe serious misdiagnosed conditions, such as:
➤ closed head injury
➤ stroke
➤ hypoglycaemia.

In addition, there are descriptions of subsequent deaths from:
➤ acute intoxication
➤ alcohol withdrawal
➤ drug toxicity
➤ overdose
➤ suicide.

Negative attitudes and beliefs by professionals are not the only determining factors. Poor clinical competence in recognising and responding to mental health–substance use conditions contribute. Other factors include overcrowding and a lack of inpatient bed access. Professionals are required, at times of peak presentation, to make decisions regarding the rationing of care and resources. These decisions are often at odds with the notion of ethically driven decision making. This leads to tension and frustration, as well as inadequate healthcare delivery.[6,16]

RACISM AND 'DESERVEDNESS OF CARE'
Racism towards Indigenous and other vulnerable groups can influence the receipt of adequate healthcare. Many are denied services due to their racial identity and substance use profile. Therefore, they are deemed by services *as not deserving* of healthcare.[17–19]

In 2006, Roche stated:

> It is increasingly recognised that a major barrier to receipt of optimal clinical care by clients with alcohol and drug-related problems is the stigma attached to these behaviours and any associated problems. The stigmatised nature of this area of work is reflected in views [of professionals] about the deservingness of clients for high quality and timely care. Yet, in spite of the common understanding of the pervasive nature of stigma in relation to alcohol and other

drug matters, relatively little systematic effort has been directed to addressing this pivotal issue.[20]

Similarly, many mental health–substance use problems resolve spontaneously, or respond to early intervention by primary health services. However, many individuals experiencing mental health–substance use concerns and dilemmas fail to receive timely services, being viewed as being morally weak and to blame for their problems. They are 'too hard' to treat, and their problems are considered to have little importance compared to 'legitimate' illnesses deserving of quality healthcare.[7,21]

BURDENS OF DISEASE

Depression is expected to be the second leading cause of disease burden in the developed world by 2020.[22] Research shows that approximately 25% of young people who present with a psychological disorder also present with a mental health–substance use problems, the most prevalent being substance use.[23] The longer-term health and economic implications of failure to address mental health–substance use problems are potentially enormous.[24]

In developing countries mental health–substance use contributes more to the overall burden of disease and disability than any other category of non-communicable disease. However, only a small minority of people affected have access to primary healthcare for these conditions.[9] In developed countries, the major issue is not health services per capita but often stigma and prejudice.[8]

SEEKING HELP

While people may seek help from specialist substance use and mental health services, they also present to general practitioners, other primary health services, and local hospitals. If incarcerated they may present to the prison medical service. These are vital opportunities to assess, diagnose and provide early interventions and referrals. Yet, people with mental health–substance use problems continue to be ignored, or actively refused care. However, stigma and prejudice are only one set of barriers to accessing proper healthcare. Another set are the ingrained expectations of the individual. Individuals often do not seek help due to:

➤ shame
➤ learned helplessness
➤ experiences of judgemental and dismissive attitudes.

Consequently, the individual may only seek help when his/her health is seriously threatened. Indeed it is often a particularly rare and brave act when help is sought prior to life-threatening crisis.

PRIMARY HEALTH SETTINGS

SELF-ASSESSMENT EXERCISE 5.1

> **Time: 45 minutes**
> Using the four case scenarios below (Joe, Kim, Brian and Sofia), write down what you feel would be a positive and helpful response(s) for each individual.
> *Compare your responses with those given in the Self-assessment exercise 5.1 answers, pp. 61–2.*

What follows offers four case scenarios that illustrate negative responses towards people seeking help in the primary healthcare setting. The positive responses can be found in Self-assessment exercise 5.1 answers, on pp. 61–2.

KEY POINT 5.2

Presenting scenarios is a powerful way to raise the key issues related to a particular incident. This illustrates what went wrong at the time, and what could go wrong in future. Issues such as:
- knowledge deficits
- skills deficits
- poor attitude
- racism
- inadequate diagnoses

need to be raised, and compared, with best practice.

Case scenario 1: Joe
Heroin

Joe has been going to the local general practice clinic for about two years. During a consultation with his regular general practitioner, Joe says that he has constipation and poor appetite. On reviewing Joe's records, the general practitioner notes that he has presented with these complaints four times over the last six months. On further questioning, Joe says he thinks this is caused by his heroin use, which has occurred regularly for about a year. Joe also says he does not want to stop using heroin as it helps with his 'problems' but he does want help for the constipation and poor appetite.[20]

Negative response

The general practitioner strongly reprimands Joe for using heroin and immediately terminates the consultation, telling him there is nothing he can do for him and to go to the drug treatment service.

Case scenario 2: Kim
Alcohol

Kim has been coming to the women's health centre for two years. During a consultation with the women's health nurse she says that she has recently been troubled by stomach pains and indigestion. On reviewing her records, the nurse notes that Kim has presented with this problem before (four times in the last six months). On close enquiry Kim says that she feels this has developed since she started drinking more. Kim says she does not wish to stop drinking and only wants her gastritis treated[20]

Negative response

The nurse tells Kim that she needs to 'get a grip' and stop drinking as this is causing the stomach pain and indigestion. She then immediately terminates the discussion.

Case scenario 3: Brian
Schizophrenia

On Monday evening, Brian presents to the emergency department. He has been feeling increasingly anxious and frightened by the command hallucinations. He is agitated, slightly sweaty and is speaking rapidly. On further questioning, the triage nurse elicits that these command hallucinations are telling Brian to harm himself. Brian denies any thought of suicidal ideation, and agrees to remain in the emergency department for assessment by the Emergency Department and Mental Health clinicians. It is busy and there are several other mental health presentations waiting for assessment. Following a wait of several hours, Brian begins pacing and muttering to himself. Upon being approached by a member of nursing staff, Brian starts talking in a loud voice and swinging his bag above his head.

Negative response

A violence response code is initiated. Brian is placed on a barouche, full limb restraints are applied and he is forced into a cubicle with a guard observing him. He continues to be distressed and thrashes about on the barouche. As a result he receives several doses of intravenous benzodiazepine. This causes him to be deeply sedated and no additional assessment of Brian is possible. Overnight, Brian awakes intermittently and requires multiple violence response team callouts due to benzodiazepine induced disinhibition. He is ultimately moved to a secure room in the psychiatric intensive care unit, where he is placed in seclusion.

Case scenario 4: Sofia
Amphetamines

On a Sunday night Sofia presents to the emergency department with heart palpitations but no chest pain. The triage nurse recognises her as she has previously presented with similar symptoms several times over the last three months. The nurse requests a medical assessment immediately. On further questioning, Sofia tells the doctor that she gets these symptoms when she has taken amphetamines. She has been doing this for about three or four months. Sofia says she does not inject but feels she cannot stop using amphetamines at the moment. She is scared that she has a serious heart problem and asks for help.[20]

Negative response

The doctor reprimands Sofia for using amphetamines saying *of course your heart is stressed'* so stop using. He also disregards her fear about her heart and refers her for a non-urgent cardiac examination. The next available appointment is in the next month or so.

SPECIALIST MENTAL HEALTH–SUBSTANCE USE SERVICES SETTINGS
'It's not our business'

Barriers to specialist mental health and substance use services exist as a direct result of mental health–substance use. This often occurs when a person's 'primary' condition, such as drug use or mental illness, is deemed not to meet the entry criteria of the particular service, from which, they seek help. Here is a scenario that illustrates this situation; it illustrates the negative responses towards Fran. The positive response(s) can be found in the Self-assessment exercise 5.2 answers, on p. 62.

SELF-ASSESSMENT EXERCISE 5.2

Time: 15 minutes
- Using Fran's case scenarios below, write down what you feel would be a positive and helpful response(s).
- Compare your responses with those given in the Self-assessment exercise 5.2 answers, p. 62.

Case scenario: Fran
Drug dependence and depression

Late Monday afternoon, Sue presents to the community mental health clinic with her flatmate, Fran. Sue tells the nurse that Fran is withdrawn, sleeps a lot and is now talking about not wanting to wake up. When questioned, Fran says she has been taking increasing amounts of painkillers and sedatives for about 18 months to stop thinking about 'what happened to her'. Fran says she needs help for her 'sadnesses', panic attacks and drug use.

Negative response

The nurse tells Fran that this service does not provide treatment for drug addiction.

Therefore, she should go to the drug unit to sort that out before coming back to the mental health clinic.

THE JUVENILE JUSTICE SYSTEM SETTING

Many young people, aged between 12 and 17 years, who are detained in the juvenile justice system experience poorer health, including mental health problems, than the general youth population. Moreover, they are at high risk of premature death, attributable to substance use and suicide.[25] Research indicates that many young people entering the juvenile justice system already require substance use treatment, yet less than half ever report receiving assessment and treatment from specialist services, or while in detention.[26]

When young people are released from detention they face immense challenges in coping adequately, especially if their mental health–substance use problems have been ignored. They have a number of immediate needs. These include:

➤ safe housing
➤ education
➤ employment
➤ positive social networks
➤ family support.

Too often these needs remain unmet, leading to increasing social and legal problems and disempowerment into adulthood.

SELF-ASSESSMENT EXERCISE 5.3

Time: 20 minutes
Based on the knowledge and understanding gained through Self-assessment exercises 5.1 and 5.2, read Fred's case scenario. Consider Fred's background then answer the questions.

- Fred is 13 years old, small for his age and seriously malnourished.
- Fred may be at risk of mental health–substance use concerns and dilemmas due to childhood trauma.
- Fred's poor school attendance, and semi-literacy, makes it difficult to understand written information and instructions.
- Fred lacks confidence in asking for help.
- Fred has serious behavioural and communication problems.
- Fred has few, if any, positive relationships with family, peers or adults.
- Fred ran away from home two months ago to escape continual physical abuse.
- Fred has been sleeping at various people's houses, or in squats, since then.
- His father has a long history of alcohol dependence and mental illness (unknown diagnosis).
1　Determine a response(s) that would help Fred with his extensive problems.
2　List the positive responses Fred would need.

Case scenario: Fred
Childhood trauma and homelessness
Fred was detained for repeated shoplifting offences and selling amphetamines, prescription drugs (codeine and morphine) and cannabis. He was due at the juvenile court the next day. Fred was homeless and would not tell police about his family or why he was 'living rough'. He was also reluctant to tell the duty nurse about his family and said he could not remember if he had ever been to a doctor or social service. He was very quiet and appeared very anxious. Following his court appearance Fred was detained in a secure juvenile justice facility for three months during which he received little emotional and psychological support or healthcare. He was discharged back to his family without supervision or follow-up and support.

Fred needed reassurance and consistent contact from a non-judgemental health professional. He also required a comprehensive psychosocial and health assessment by an experienced professional to identify his immediate and longer-term needs. However, these responses were denied.

REFLECTIVE PRACTICE EXERCISE 5.1

Time: 30 minutes
Having read Fred's case scenario, spend some time reflecting on the following:
- Were Fred's human rights met?
  - How do you know?
  - Why might this occur?
- What impact could there have been on Fred's current and future life experiences?
- What should have been done?
- When and by whom?
- What would you have done?
- Why?

CRITICAL INCIDENTS
Recent incidents in South Australian country areas were identified through the critical incident alert system used by all public hospitals and other healthcare units. Two such cases are presented below, each confirmed by the specialist drug and alcohol nurses who were aware of each case. One of the men was Aboriginal, and both were young adults. The two incidents are presented as scenarios below, with some key interventions described that were implemented to prevent further incidences in these settings.

REFLECTIVE PRACTICE EXERCISE 5.2

Time: 20 minutes
Read Kevin's case scenario below. What would you do?

Case scenario: Kevin
Alcohol withdrawal

Kevin was a 23-year-old Aboriginal man who presented as prearranged to the local hospital for his first planned alcohol detoxification prior to his rehabilitation programme. Kevin was admitted to the medical ward as previously arranged by his general practitioner.

Day 1

On admission his blood alcohol concentration was 0.2 (mass of pure alcohol per volume of blood, e.g. blood alcohol concentration of 0.05 per cent indicates 0.05 grams of alcohol in every 100 millilitres of blood).[27] The registered nurse responsible for Kevin failed to implement the appropriate diazepam and thiamine medication regime as ordered by Kevin's general practitioner. She did not conduct a proper nursing and substance use history. She did not instigate baseline observations and regular monitoring for emerging symptoms of alcohol withdrawal as is standard practice. In particular, she did not use the Clinical Instrument Withdrawal Assessment of Alcohol Scale, Revised (CIWA-Ar), an alcohol withdrawal monitoring instrument, considered the 'gold standard' in Australia.[28]

Day 2

Kevin's withdrawal symptoms progressed alarmingly and he subsequently developed delirium tremens. He required emergency medical evacuation by helicopter to an intensive care unit. The nearest facility was 200 kilometres away in a major metropolitan hospital. Fortunately, he survived, but as a consequence of local hospital mismanagement he required a metropolitan hospital stay of two weeks.

The receiving hospital subsequently submitted a critical incident alert report to the Department of Health, which then triggered a full investigation into this serious incident. Nursing staff from the country hospital in which Kevin was originally admitted were interviewed about the poor quality of their care. They were informed that they had not undertaken the expected standards of care.

They had not instigated the CIWA-Ar alcohol withdrawal monitoring procedures or administered the prescribed medication regimes ordered by Kevin's general practitioner. Their response to this feedback was recorded to be: *'So what – he's only an Aboriginal'.*

Strategies to prevent future incidents

The local specialist drug and alcohol nurse was aware of the incident. With support of her clinical manager, she took immediate action. She contacted the hospital management and advised them of the racism that had occurred, which was unethical and unacceptable. She also advised management both in writing and in person of the poor standards of nursing care that had occurred. She and her clinical manager then assisted them in reviewing and upgrading relevant policies and protocols. The hospital management's attention was drawn to a series of freely available evidence-based clinical guidelines for nurses. These had been previously provided to all public hospitals in the state.[29]

Outcomes

All nursing and allied health staff of the hospital undertook cultural respect workshops facilitated by Aboriginal leaders. The hospital medical and nursing procedures for alcohol withdrawal observations, monitoring and treatment were immediately reviewed. They were then amended to reflect standard clinical procedures and medical regimes for alcohol withdrawal.

Use of the 'best practice' CIWA-Ar alcohol withdrawal monitoring tool, standing orders and guidelines for safe nursing care were implemented across the hospital. The drug and alcohol nurse provided training to all nursing staff on this tool. Consultation and informal nurse to nurse education and support were established. Clear referral pathways to specialist drug and alcohol and mental health services were put in place. As part of their professional development activities, nurses were required to use standard clinical guidelines during case reviews to reflect on practice and problem solve as a team.[29] In addition, anti-racism and ethical practices were discussed, and applied to case reviews.

REFLECTIVE PRACTICE EXERCISE 5.3

> **Time: 20 minutes**
> Read Peter's case scenario below. What would you do?

Case scenario: Peter
Bipolar disorder
Peter had recently been discharged from the psychiatric ward in the local hospital following his first episode of bipolar disorder. Peter reported using cannabis, amphetamines and alcohol from time to time leading up to his admission.

On discharge he had been prescribed and commenced on an anti-psychotic medication and mood stabiliser. He was referred to the local community mental health service. His case was allocated to an enrolled nurse rather than a registered psychiatric nurse. The enrolled nurse then saw Peter for five minutes at each of six occasions, fortnightly.

Peter raised various concerns about his diagnosis and treatment and asked the enrolled nurse to advise him. However, she avoided his questions. After about 12 weeks Peter was discharged from the mental health service and referred to the community drug and alcohol nurse for his alcohol, cannabis and amphetamine use. The mental health service had documented this use as being linked to his first episode of mania.

The community drug and alcohol nurse identified serious deficits in all aspects of Peter's mental health treatment. These included:

➤ no ongoing assessment
➤ no monitoring
➤ no appropriate intervention.

Peter was not having regular monitoring of his:
➤ medications
➤ weight
➤ nutritional status
➤ symptom management.

His weight had increased rapidly by 20 kilograms. His sodium valproate blood levels had not been monitored and these were elevated. Peter had complained of serious, known medication side-effects including:
➤ akasthisia
➤ light sensitivity
➤ dizziness
➤ headaches
➤ poor memory.

Peter was also worried that he may not be using his medications as prescribed due to his insomnia and subsequent sleeping late in the morning.

The mental health team had not developed an ongoing plan with Peter for early recognition and relapse prevention and management. Neither was he educated about his diagnosis and the links he could make with local self-help groups.

Peter's other concerns were his strained relationships with his family due to his recent mania. He felt they needed support and education about his condition, but these too were neglected. His family was uninformed about his condition, did not know what to expect and did not know what supports existed for them. Peter had also become socially isolated because he believed his friends would think he was 'mental', and this led to increasing reluctance to leave his house. In addition, Peter had requested that his diagnosis not be written on his medical certificate as he feared this could prevent him from getting employment, but this was ignored.

Strategy to prevent future incidents
The drug and alcohol nurse, together with her clinical manager, successfully advocated for and organised a telemedicine meeting. The meeting included an appropriate city-based psychiatrist, local mental health manager and herself. The psychiatrist recommended that Peter's anti-psychotic medication be immediately reduced by 10 mg, and then progressively ceased. The psychiatrist also recommended that blood monitoring of his sodium valproate begin immediately and be undertaken regularly. It was decided that Peter be readmitted to the community mental health team for:
➤ regular monitoring
➤ medication review
➤ health review
➤ appropriate support.

Collaboration between the mental health team and drug and alcohol nurse was considered essential to assist Peter to safely manage his mental health and alcohol and other drug use.

Despite the discussions in the telemedicine review the community mental health team manager ignored the agreed outcomes. With much frustration the drug and alcohol nurse reported this to her clinical manager. Together, they wrote a detailed case study to present the key issues to the mental health team manager and other staff. As a result meetings were held between them to design and implement a number of strategies.

Outcomes

The drug and alcohol nurse eventually successfully implemented the telemedicine recommendations and thus addressed Peter's needs and concerns. These included education for Peter and his family about his condition, medications and future management plan. It also involved linking his family members with local support groups, providing them with relevant literature, relevant websites and 24 hour telephone services should they require urgent assistance or information. The drug and alcohol nurse also educated and supported Peter on how to self-monitor his condition with good early outcomes.

New procedures for effective cross-agency cooperation and shared care were implemented. These involved a greater uptake of evidence-based approaches in person management and responses to the needs of people with mental health–substance use problems. The mental health team leader and staff all undertook formal mental health–substance use education. They were made cognisant of anti-discrimination principles and the need for this to be reflected in their practice. These strategies have since been successfully implemented by a partnership between drug and alcohol and mental health services in other country regions.

DISCUSSION

The cases presented illustrate how discrimination places people with mental health–substance use problems at serious risk. Coronial, police and critical incident reports all suggest that stereotyping, racism and unethical practices among some professionals contribute to:

➤ avoidable suffering
➤ exacerbation of physical and mental health problems
➤ prolonged hospitalisation
➤ disenfranchisement from society
➤ premature disability and death.

In particular, the critical incident reports identified that inexcusable discrimination and unethical clinical practices on the part of individuals were not the only determining factor. At fault were the inappropriate or inadequate organisational management, policies and protocols of these services.

A particularly effective strategy in assisting organisational commitment to change has been when professionals have presented relevant case studies to senior management of the facilities, in which the incidents occur. This provides the opportunity for professionals to be informed and able to discuss the individual's clinical condition, and various interventions, objectively. From these discussions, the professionals can be engaged in mutual problem solving, leading to the development and implementation of evidence-based:

➤ policies
➤ practices
➤ safer responses
➤ quality health and psychosocial care.

As a supporting mechanism drug and alcohol nurses can offer flexible education to meet the needs of clinicians and organisations. This may consist of 'bedside' mentoring of hospital and community mental health nurses. They can also facilitate the use of evidence-based clinical guidelines, medication regimes and reliable instruments.[29] This has worked well where local organisational leaders and clinicians have responded positively to the issues and need for change. However, these strategies cannot be effective when organisational leaders and clinicians continue to allow racism and denial of healthcare for people with mental health–substance use problems.

It is always important to try to redress situations at the 'ground level'. Meetings with service managers should focus on quality improvement relating to critical incidents. The focus needs to be on the:
➤ situation
➤ risks
➤ deficits in service delivery
➤ what needs to be improved.

Presenting scenarios is a powerful way to raise the key issues related to a particular incident as this illustrates what went wrong at the time, and what could go wrong in the future. Issues, such as:
➤ knowledge deficits
➤ skills deficits
➤ poor attitudes
➤ racism
➤ inadequate diagnoses
➤ all need to be raised and compared with best practice.

KEY POINT 5:3

Key recommendations for consideration
All health services, wherever they are, should reflect the 2008 National Mental Health Policy in Australia which aims: 'to assure the rights of people with mental health problems and mental illness, and enable them to participate meaningfully in society',[30] and the National Drug Strategy 2004–2009 which aims to 'increase access to a greater range of high-quality prevention and treatment services'.[31]
Some ways in which these aims can be met locally are through good governance and clinical practices within health services including the following.
1 Racism and judgemental attitudes and behaviours by any staff towards people with mental health–substance use concerns and dilemmas are zero-tolerated.
2 Evidence-based policies, protocols and guidelines are implemented in all hospitals and health units to ensure appropriate assessment, treatment and support for people with mental health–substance use concerns and dilemmas.

3 Regular training on delivering culturally respectful services is provided to all relevant health professionals, including first point of contact clerical staff, to ensure competence in delivering non-discriminatory services to all individuals, at all times.

4 Effective collaboration cross-agency (intra- and interdisciplinary) teamwork for people with mental health-substance use concerns and dilemmas is planned for, and implemented, effectively.

5 Critical incident reporting systems are monitored, and acted on, so that no person is refused healthcare based on their race or presumed mental health–substance use concerns and dilemmas.

6 Regular clinical supervision and case reviews are undertaken so that all clinicians reflect on their practice by discussing case presentations and debriefing in a collegial and supportive environment.

7 All professionals have access to freely available evidence-based clinical guidelines (*see* reference 29).

CONCLUSION

Denial of people's right to safe healthcare for mental health–substance use problems is unethical and unsafe. However, it still occurs from a complex interaction of systemic factors, including:

➤ inappropriate or absence of organisational policy
➤ poor management and leadership
➤ unsafe behaviours of health professionals.

These factors are condoned, or ignored, by organisations and professions. These unacceptable influences are at times based on:

➤ stigmatisation of people with mental health–substance use problems
➤ racism.

Effective and urgent action to redress this situation is needed at all levels of healthcare governance, policy and healthcare practice.

POST-READING EXERCISE 5.1

Time: 30 minutes
In Pre-reading exercise 5.1 you were asked to consider the following 'An individual is offered substandard, or no, healthcare because of his/her race or presenting health problem(s).

● How could this situation impact on this individual?
● How would you advocate for him/her?
● What might stop you from advocating for him/her?
● What would enable you to advocate for him/her?

Revisit your conclusions and reflect:
What more do you know about the impact on the individual?

● What else could you do now when advocating for the individual?

- What would stop you?
- What would enable you?

REFERENCES

1 World Health Organization. *Constitution of the World Health Organization*. TFWH Assembly; 2006. Available at: www.who.int/governance/eb/who_constitution_en.pdf (accessed 9 March 2010).

2 Thompson A, Putnins A. Risk-need assessment inventories for juvenile offenders in Australia. *Psychiatry, Psychology and Law*. 2003; **10**: 324–33.

3 Wilson A. Planning primary health-care services for South Australian young offenders: a preliminary study. *Int J Nurs Pract*. 2007; **13**: 296–303.

4 de Crespigny C. Double jeopardy: disadvantage and drug problems. *Aust J Prim Health*. 2002; **8**: 70–6.

5 de Crespigny C, Emden C, Drage B, *et al*. Missed opportunities in the field: caring for clients with co-morbidity problems. *Collegian*. 2002; **9**: 29–34.

6 Stuhlmiller C, Tolchard B, Thomas L, *et al*. Increasing confidence of emergency department staff in responding to mental illness: an educational initiative. *AENJ*. 2004; **7**: 9–17.

7 Skinner N, Feather N, Freeman T, *et al*. Stigma and discrimination in health care provision to drug users: the role of values, affect and deservingness judgments. *J Appl Soc Psychol*. 2007; **37**: 163–86.

8 Talmet J, de Crespigny C, Cusack, L, *et al*. 'Turning a blind eye': denying people their right to treatment for acute alcohol, drug and mental health conditions – an act of discrimination. *Ment Health Subst Use*. 2009; **2**: 247–54.

9 Ban Ki-Moon, Secretary-General. *Secretary-General lays out challenging UN agenda for 2008*. United Nations News Centre, United Nations; 2008. Available at: www.un.org/apps/news/story. asp?NewsID=27164&Cr=drug&Cr1 (accessed 2 September 2010); United Nations. *The Universal Declaration of Human Rights: a living document*. Available at: www.healthwrights.org/static/nl44-charter.PDF (accessed 2 September 2010).

10 Chowdhury Z, Rowson M. The people's health assembly. *BMJ*. **321**: 1361–2.

11 Wayne Chivell, Coroner. [Findings of Inquest for Jarrod Stonehouse.] Adelaide, SA: 2000. Available at: www.courts.sa.gov.au/courts/coroner/findings/findings_2000/stonehouse.finding. htm (accessed 9 March 2010).

12 AustLII Joint Facility of University of Technology Sydney and University of New South Wales Faculties of Law. Australian Indigenous Law Library. Available at: www.austlii.edu.au/au/special/ indigenous (accessed 9 March 2010).

13 Kalucy R, Thomas L, King D. Changing demand for mental health services in the emergency department of a public hospital. *Aust N Z J Psychiatry*. 2005; **39**: 74–80.

14 Knott JC, Pleban A, Taylor, D, *et al*. Management of mental health patients attending Victorian emergency departments. *Aust N Z J Psychiatry*. 2007; **41**: 759–67.

15 Wand T, White K. Exploring the scope of the Emergency Department mental health nurse practitioner role. *Int J Ment Health Nurs*. 2007; **16**: 403–12.

16 de Crespigny C, Kowanko I, Murray H, *et al*. A nursing partnership for better outcomes in Aboriginal alcohol, other drugs and mental health. *Contemp Nurse*. 2006; **22**: 257–87

17 de Crespigny C, Groenkjaer M, Casey W, *et al*. Racism and injustice: urban Aboriginal women's experiences when patronising licensed premises in South Australia. *Aust J Prim Health*. 2003; **9**: 111–17.

18 de Crespigny C, Emden C, Murray H. A partnership model for ethical indigenous research. *Collegian*. 2004; **11**: 17–18.

19 Kowanko I, de Crespigny C, Murray H. *Better Medication Management for Aboriginal People with Mental Health Disorders and their Carers. Final Report.* Adelaide, SA: Flinders University; 2003.

20 National Centre for Education and Training on Addiction. *Health Professionals' Attitudes Towards Licit and Illicit Drug Users: a training resource.* Adelaide, SA: National Centre for Education and Training on Addiction; 2006. pp. 7–9.

21 Featherstone N, Johnstone C. Social norms, entitlement and deservingness: differential reactions to aggressive behaviour of schizophrenic and personality disorder patients. *Pers Soc Psychol Bull.* 2001; **27**: 755–67.

22 Lopez AD, Murray CC. The global burden of disease, 1990–2020. *Nat Med.* 1998; **4**: 1241–3.

23 Teesson M, Hall W, Lynskey M, *et al.* The epidemiology of drug dependence in Australia: findings from the National Survey of Mental Health and Wellbeing. *Problems of Drug Dependence 1999: Proceedings of the 61st Annual Scientific Meeting, the College on Problems of Drug Dependence.* National Institute of Drug Abuse (NIDA), Research Monograph 180; 2000. Available at www.med.unsw.edu.au/NDARCWeb.nsf/page/External%20Publications (accessed 9 March 2010).

24 Goren N, Mallick J. Prevention and early intervention of coexisting mental health and substance use issues: *Prevention Research Quarterly: Issues Paper.* Australian Drug Foundation. 2007; **3**. Available at: www.druginfo.adf.org.au/downloads/Prevention_Research_Quarterly/IP_No2_07_Prev_sub_abuse_mentalhealth.pdf (accessed 9 March 2010).

25 Coffey C, Veit F, Wolfe R, *et al.* Mortality in young offenders: retrospective cohort study. *BMJ.* 2003; **326**: 1064.

26 Johnson TP, Cho YI, Fendrich M, *et al.* Treatment need and utilization among youth entering the juvenile corrections system. *J Subst Abuse Treat.* 2004; **26**(2): 117–28.

27 Drug and Alcohol Services of South Australia (DASSA). *Blood Alcohol Concentration (BAC).* Adelaide, SA: Drug and Alcohol Services of South Australia; 2008.

28 Sullivan JT, Sykora K, Schneiderman J, *et al.* Assessment of alcohol withdrawal: the revised clinical institute withdrawal assessment for alcohol scale (CIWA-Ar). *Br J Addict.* 1989; **84**: 1353–7.

29 de Crespigny C, Talmet J, Modystack K, *et al. Alcohol Tobacco and other Drugs: clinical guidelines for nurses and midwives. Version 2.* Adelaide, SA: School of Nursing and Midwifery, Flinders University; 2003.

30 Commonwealth of Australia. *Mental Health Policy 2008. National Mental Health Strategy.* Canberra, ACT: Commonwealth of Australia; 2009. p. 2.

31 Ministerial Council on Drugs. *The National Drug Strategy Australia's Integrated Framework 2004–2009. Ministerial Council on Drug Strategy.* Canberra, ACT: Commonwealth of Australia; 2004. p. 5.

TO LEARN MORE

Allsop S. *Drug Use and Mental Health: effective responses to co-occurring drug and mental health problems.* Melbourne, VIC: IP Communications; 2008.

Baker A, Velleman R. *Clinical Handbook of Co-existing Mental Health and Drug and Alcohol Problems.* London and New York: Routledge; 2007.

Couzos S, Murray R. *Aboriginal Primary Health Care.* 3rd ed. Melbourne, VIC: Oxford University Press; 2008.

McMurray A. *Community Health and Wellness: a socio-ecological approach.* 3rd ed. Marrickville, NSW: Elsevier; 2007.

EXERCISE ANSWERS

SELF-ASSESSMENT EXERCISE 5.1 ANSWERS: POSITIVE RESPONSES

Having prepared your positive responses to the four case scenarios on pp. 48–50, compare your responses with the positive responses given below. What have you learnt? What is similar? What is different? What can you do in your work environment?

Case scenario 1: Joe

The general practitioner gives Joe information on heroin effects, preventing overdose, safe injecting practices and how pharmacotherapy might be useful at some stage. She encourages Joe to make another appointment for an extended consultation the following day so they can:

- undertake a physical and mental health assessment and substance use history
- discuss how to best manage his heroin use
- monitor his mood and, if required, treat his depression
- ensure Joe knows that he is supported in getting drug treatment and general healthcare at any time.[20]

Case scenario 2: Kim

The nurse responds to Kim by assuring her that she can be helped. The nurse begins by suggesting further assessment by the doctor to identify what is causing the gastritis symptoms, and makes an appointment for the next day. She also offers Kim information about alcohol effects on the body, good nutrition including vitamin and mineral supplements, and in particular vitamin B[1] (thiamine). The nurse then encourages Kim to make another appointment for an extended consultation to discuss:

- Kim's general issues
- conduct a mental health and substance use history
- reducing her drinking to a level she feels she can manage
- increasing her understanding of how drinking problems can be treated if, and when, she is ready to change.[20]

Case scenario 3: Brian

The triage nurse identifies Brian's increasing agitation and increases his triage priority. Brian is moved into a cubicle and is assessed by an appropriately skilled nurse. This assessment includes both a physical and mental health assessment. It is discovered that Brian has recently been diagnosed with schizophrenia. The initial assessment by the emergency department clinician reveals that there is no underlying medical pathology and that Brian is experiencing an acute psychotic episode. He is deemed to be at risk to himself and is detained under the Mental Health Act. A rapid-acting atypical antipsychotic is administered. This results in Brian being slightly sedated. He is placed on half-hourly visual observations and awaits the review of the mental health team registrar with a view to being admitted to an inpatient mental health facility.[20]

Case scenario 4: Sofia

The triage nurse requests that Sofia has an immediate cardiac assessment. Once admitted to a hospital ward and her medical treatment has been initiated Sofia:

- receives a full mental health and substance use assessment
- is offered social work follow-up and counselling to support her
- is provided with information about drug treatment and support services should she decide she is ready to cease her amphetamine use.[20]

SELF-ASSESSMENT EXERCISE 5.2 ANSWERS: POSITIVE RESPONSES

Having prepared your positive responses to Fran's case scenarios on p. 50 compare your responses with the positive responses given below. What have you learnt? What is similar? What is different? What can you do in your work environment?

Case scenario: Fran

The nurse reassures Fran that she can be helped and, with her permission, immediately makes arrangements for her admission to the mental health inpatient unit. She explains to Fran that she will receive a full assessment (drug history, mental and physical health examination) and that her drug withdrawal would be managed symptomatically. She will also receive support and treatment for her panicky feelings and 'sadnesses'. She reassures Fran that she will be safe and in a welcoming environment with staff who have genuine concern for her welfare and expertise to help her.

CHAPTER 6

The importance of physical health assessment

John R Ashcroft

PRE-READING EXERCISE 6.1

Time: 10 minutes
Starting from head and working down, brainstorm the physical consequences of substance use (alcohol, drugs and tobacco).
Compare your list with the answers to Pre-reading exercise 6.1 on p. 77.

INTRODUCTION

When addressing mental health–substance use, there can be a tendency to omit the imperative assessment of physical health. This chapter looks at some physical health antecedents and consequences. However, it is not exhaustive and the reader is directed to the 'To learn more' section within this chapter, the 'Useful chapters' section of this book, and encouraged to take up his/her own learning programme.

Physical health assessment in mental health–substance use is more than simply physical examination or routine screening that occurs upon initial entry into the caring services. Rather, it is an ongoing process reflective of the needs of the individual. The relationship between physical health, mental health and substance use is complex. The behaviour, and the physical and mental health of an individual, greatly influence, and are influenced by, the environment and social circumstances. In addition to the importance of recognising and treating physical problems, it is acknowledged that poor physical and mental health can influence behaviour and contribute to substance use (*see* Figure 6.1).

Users of illicit substances typically live a chaotic lifestyle, often repeatedly engaging in risk-taking behaviour. It is the repetitive nature of substance use behaviour, and the chaos that can ensue, which requires an *ongoing* physical health assessment.

KEY POINT 6.1

Comprehensive physical health assessment is an ongoing dynamic process.

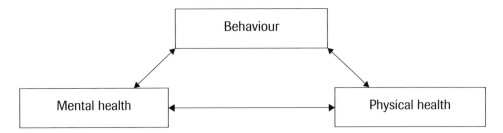

FIGURE 6.1 Drug and alcohol use (behaviour) may contribute to deterioration in both mental and physical health which may then contribute to further substance use

HEALTHY BODY – HEALTHY MIND

It is accepted that good physical health promotes psychological well-being. The better we feel mentally, the more likely we are to try to remain physically well. However, the converse is also true. Poor physical health may contribute to poor mental health. Moreover, psychological disturbance may further impact on physical health through poor lifestyle choices in an attempt to alleviate subjective distress (*see* Figure 6.2). Coping strategies often include the use of alcohol, tobacco and substances.[1]

> **KEY POINT 6.2**
>
> The individual with mental ill health tends to be in poorer physical health and has an increased risk of mortality from both natural and unnatural causes.[2,3,4]

An appreciation of the potential contribution of psychological symptoms, or psychiatric ill health, to physical disease, highlights the need for neuropsychiatric evaluation as part of comprehensive physical health screening and assessment. Indeed, inclusion of mental health assessment in physical health assessment is not unique to the specialty of substance use. For example, there is evidence to suggest that depression may be an independent risk factor for heart disease in men,[5] *'an association independent of smoking status, diabetes, hypertension and deprivation score'*.[5] Other studies suggest an association between chronic anxiety and peptic ulcers.[6] Therefore, treatment of symptoms of anxiety and depression (pharmacologically or psychotherapeutically) may potentially decrease the risk of heart disease, and peptic ulcer disease, respectively. Similarly, the treatment of physical disease and psychological disturbance in people with substance use problems may be influential in terms of management of the substance use.

> **KEY POINT 6.3**
>
> 'You never really understand a person until you consider things from his point of view . . . until you climb into his skin and walk around in it.'[7]

Given that the physical, mental and social aspects of life are often closely interconnected, an eclectic, holistic, person-centred approach to assessment is essential.

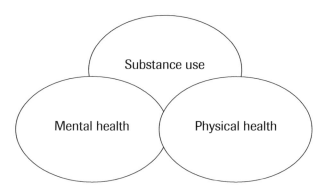

FIGURE 6.2 Drug and alcohol use is associated with an increase of physical health problems leading to significant comorbidity

An understanding and appreciation of this connection is paramount if measures are to be in place to improve quality of life.

SELF-ASSESSMENT EXERCISE 6.1

Time: 10 minutes
Consider the following scenario; what would you observe?
Sarah is a 34-year-old sex worker who, despite currently being prescribed methadone, continues to inject heroin daily into her groin. Sarah was recently found to be HIV positive. Since learning of her HIV status, Sara has become extremely depressed in mood, experiencing suicidal thoughts. Sarah's sleep and appetite are poor, and she has lost several stone in weight. Her alcohol use has greatly increased. Sara has returned to the use of crack cocaine. Urine screen today suggests she is pregnant.

In the above case scenario, Sarah's *behaviour* (injecting heroin and prostitution) is likely to have resulted in her acquiring HIV (*physical health*), and a deterioration in her *mental health*. The consequent low mood and suicidal thoughts appear to have contributed to an increase in Sarah's substance use *behaviour* and a further deterioration in her *physical health*.

Under normal circumstances Sarah's pregnancy would not be viewed as pathological. However, in this case there would be serious concerns about the potential impact upon both her physical and mental well-being. For Sarah, an assessment that focused on her HIV status or pregnancy alone would be incomplete. Therefore, an understanding of how issues have come together, and the consequent effects upon her psychological well-being, is required if attempts are to be made to break the cycle (*see* Figure 6.1).

THE PRINCIPAL AIMS OF PHYSICAL HEALTH SCREENING AND ASSESSMENT

KEY POINT 6.4

The use of two or more substances greatly increases the risk of physical health problems and overdose.[7]

There are six principal aims of screening and assessment as follows.

1 To identify existing physical and mental health problems
The physical consequences of substance use may be directly related to the biological or physiological effects on the body, or associated with the means of administration of the substance(s) (*see* Table 6.1).

TABLE 6.1 Means of administration and possible physical complications associated

Means of administration	Associated physical health complications
Injection	• Sharing blood-contaminated equipment (needles and pipes) increases the risk of acquiring blood-borne virus infections (hepatitis A, B, C and HIV) • Pain, swelling and bruising at injection site • Risk of tetanus • Staphylococcal and streptococcal infections may lead to cellulitis, abscesses, ulceration, septicaemia, bacterial endocarditis • Deep venous thrombosis and pulmonary embolism • Increased risk of overdose
Smoking and inhalation	• Chest infections, bronchitis, haemoptysis, chronic obstructive pulmonary disease, carcinoma of the lung • Inhalation of aerosols is associated with cardiac arrhythmias and may cause sudden death
Insufflation (Snorting)	• Necrosis of the nasal septum
Oral consumption	• Tooth decay, gastritis, oesophagitis

TABLE 6.2 Drug combinations and potential pharmacological interactions

Drug combination	Potential consequence
Opiates and benzodiazepines	Sedation, risk of respiratory depression and overdose
Opiates and tricyclic antidepressants	Sedation, risk of respiratory depression and overdose

(*continued*)

Drug combination	Potential consequence
Alcohol and central nervous system depressants (opiates, benzodiazepines, tricyclic antidepressants)	Sedation, risk of respiratory depression and overdose, hypotension
Opiates and anticonvulsants	Plasma concentration of methadone reduced by carbamazepine and phenytoin possibly leading to withdrawal symptoms
Heroin (or other opiate) followed by buprenorphine	Risk of precipitated withdrawal symptoms
Buprenorphine followed by heroin (or other opiate)	Attempt to overcome the blockade effect of buprenorphine could result in overdose
Lofexidine and anxiolytics/hypnotics	Increased sedative effect
Naltrexone and opiate-based analgesia (cocodamol, codydramol)	Blocks analgesic effect. Attempt to overcome blockade could result in opiate overdose

The physical consequence of opiate use is often related to the mode of administration. However, if taken in sufficient quantities or with other medication (*see* Table 6.2) there is significant risk of accidental overdose and death. Similarly to opiates, stimulants (cocaine, amphetamines) may be administered in several ways. They act systemically to increase blood pressure and heart rate and consequently may cause arrhythmias,[8] myocardial infarction[9] and stroke.[10,11]

Heavy alcohol consumption is associated with considerable health problems affecting multiple organs and systems in the body.[12] Gastrointestinal complications include:
➤ gastritis
➤ peptic ulcer disease
➤ alcoholic hepatitis
➤ cirrhosis.

Cardiovascular complications include:
➤ hypertension
➤ arrhythmias.

Although light to moderate alcohol consumption may be associated with a lower risk of coronary heart disease, high consumption is associated with an increased risk. Long-term use is associated with carcinoma of the:
➤ mouth
➤ oesophagus
➤ colon
➤ liver.[13]

The neurological complications of prolonged heavy alcohol consumption may be associated with a variety of neuropsychiatric symptoms including:
➤ anxiety
➤ depression
➤ psychosis.

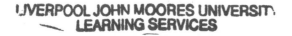

Assessment of substance use should not be overlooked. Moreover, it is important to screen and assess for conditions not directly related to substance use.

> ### KEY POINTS 6.5
>
> Users of drugs and alcohol are less likely to seek help for physical symptoms.
> If medical attention is sought, it is possible that the symptoms will be attributed to lifestyle and substance use rather than unrelated pathology.
>   This may cause unnecessary delay in treatment and further deterioration in physical health.

Self-neglect, in the form of poor nourishment (spending money on substance use rather than food), and poor compliance with recommended diet or prescribed medication, is a concern.
    Comorbid conditions, such as
➤ diabetes mellitus
➤ hypertension
➤ thyroid disorders
➤ epilepsy

may be poorly managed, increasing the risk of disease complications. Moreover, the screening and assessment process may identify such problems in the previously unaware individual.

Individuals who use substances are at particular risk of exacerbation of pre-existing respiratory conditions, or the development of chronic disease secondary to smoke inhalation. Conditions such as asthma and chronic obstructive pulmonary disease should be managed appropriately.

Head and brain injury
A complex relationship exists between brain injury and substance use. Alcohol and drug use may precede brain injury, and intoxication is often implicated in brain trauma secondary to accident or assault.[13] The substances used may cause brain damage directly by means of neurotoxicity, cerebral ischaemia or infarction (i.e. direct causes). In addition, brain damage may result indirectly (indirect causes) by means of vitamin deficiency (Wernicke–Korsakoff syndrome),[14] or hepatic impairment (hepatic encephalopathy).[15]
    Substance use may occur following brain injury for a variety of reasons (including a means of self-medication, or simply recreational use), and contribute to further brain injury. In this way, a substance use–brain injury cycle may develop, potentially with a progressive deterioration in cognitive function (*see* Figure 6.3).

Mental health screening and assessment
Mental health screening and assessment may identify psychiatric ill health and psychological symptoms, possibly amenable to pharmacological and psychological treatment.

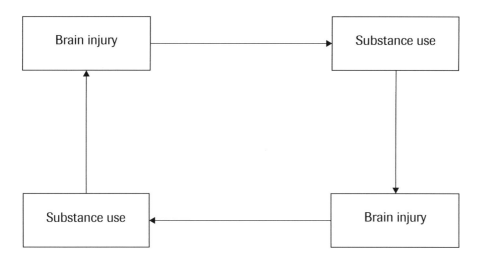

FIGURE 6.3 Substance use–brain injury cycle

Screening and assessment provide an opportunity to review the existing plan of care for the person with a previously diagnosed mental ill health who may already be prescribed medication.

KEY POINT 6.6

Be alert to the need to liaise/involve mental health, physical health and specialist substance use services.

Psychological disturbance may be related to intoxication, or a reaction to adverse social conditions associated with substance use. Moreover, substance use may exacerbate pre-existing mental health problems, and interact with prescribed medication. Psychotic symptoms may be deemed 'drug induced' if they persist beyond the period of acute intoxication, and can be distinguished from primary mental ill health.

Mental ill health may be precipitated by substance use in the person predisposed genetically.[17] It should be recocognised that the neuropsychiatric manifestations evident, following prolonged substance use, may be reflective of brain damage and the processes described above (i.e the indirect and direct causal processes).

2 To identify those at risk of physical ill health and put measures in place to minimise the risks

Although eradication of risk-taking behaviour and abstinence from substances may be the individuals chosen goal of treatment, measures can be put in place to minimise the risk of future ill health. In addition to the person already diagnosed with physical ill health, measures may be put in place to prevent, or slow, further deterioration, or indeed to treat or return to previous health norms.

SELF-ASSESSMENT EXERCISE 6.2

Time: 5 minutes
List what education may be offered to the person who uses substances.

Sharing paraphernalia
Education about the risks of sharing equipment (needles, pipes, spoons), and providing information of the availability of needle exchange programmes is crucial to the prevention of the spread of blood-borne viruses. Moreover, such programmes help avoid tissue trauma and the contraction of tetanus caused by the reuse of blunt and dirty needles.

Sexual health
Individuals who use substances may be referred to specialist services. Individuals at highest risk of sexually transmitted diseases (particularly sex workers) may be offered advice about safe sex practices and referred to genito-urinary medicine. In addition, information about contraception, referrals made to family planning clinics, and cervical smears can be arranged for the person at risk. Substance use is associated with infertility in both men and women and is often secondary to hormonal imbalance. Therefore, treatment often leads to improved fertility.

Vaccinations are available for hepatitis A and B. However, although vaccinations are not available for hepatitis C and HIV, they are preventable. Combination treatment with pegylated interferon and ribavirin is available for the treatment of hepatitis C, although success in clearing the virus varies according to stage of disease and genotype. In the person diagnosed with HIV disease, progression may be slowed by combinations of antiretroviral drugs.[1]

Tobacco use
Many people smoke cigarettes, although often this is not addressed. Smoking cessation may reduce the risk of respiratory conditions, although there may also be some evidence to suggest that it is associated with improved treatment outcomes.[19]

3 Consideration and implementation of pharmacological intervention
Prescribed drugs have side-effects, cautions, contraindications and potential interactions with other substances (prescribed and non-prescribed). The decision to prescribe medication requires an understanding of the biological and physiological effect of a drug on the body (pharmacodynamics). In addition, knowledge of the way in which the body metabolises and excretes the drug (pharmacokinetics) is essential. Pharmacodynamics and pharmacokinetics are greatly influenced by:
➤ the physical health of the individual receiving the drug
➤ other medication prescribed.

This highlights the importance of physical health screening and assessment.

Drugs are eliminated from the body following a process of metabolism in the liver (where lipid-soluble drugs are metabolised to more water-soluble compounds), and renal excretion. Water-soluble drugs are generally excreted unchanged in the kidney.

Hepatic and renal impairment may greatly influence the excretion of a number of drug classes and baseline blood tests are recommended.

Several combinations of drug classes pose particular risks (*see* Table 6.2). Essentially, there is an increased risk of sedation, respiratory depression, coma and death when sedative drugs are prescribed together. The risk is substantially increased when used in combination with alcohol and/or illicit substances (e.g. non-prescribed benzodiazepines, buprenorphine or methadone and heroin). In addition, drugs may influence the metabolism of a concurrently prescribed drug, leading to the prescription of higher or lower doses than usually necessary.

Anticonvulsant drugs, such as carbamazepine and phenytoin, induce liver enzymes and may lead to a reduction in the plasma concentration of methadone. A higher dose than normally required may need to be prescribed to overcome withdrawal symptoms. However, abrupt discontinuation of anticonvulsant medication may lead to a rise in plasma methadone levels, and its central nervous system (CNS) depressant effect. Therefore, it may be necessary to alter doses accordingly.

> **KEY POINT 6.7**
>
> It is imparative that good communication exists between professionals to ensure safe prescribing.

The choice of form of the particular drug may be influenced by the physical health of the individual. Liquid preparations may be preferred to tablets – where swallowing difficulties are present – and sugar-free methadone offered to the individual with poor dental hygiene or diabetes mellitus. Inability to chew food may contribute to weight loss and further deterioration in physical health.

Drugs typically prescribed in the substance use setting
OPIATE SUBSTITUTION (METHADONE OR BUPRENORPHINE)
The National Institute for Health and Clinical Excellence (NICE)[20] recommends the prescription of either methadone or buprenorphine for the management of opioid dependence. However, when combined with other central nervous system depressant medication (*see* Table 6.2), the risk of overdose is significantly increased.

Methadone is metabolised by the liver and excreted by the kidneys into the urine. Hepatic, or renal, impairment may increase its bioavailability and consequently increasing the risk of overdose. Liver function test and kidney function tests (urea and electrolytes) may be used to guide the:
➤ initial prescribed dose
➤ titration rate of methadone
➤ decision to adjust the dose already prescribed.

Methadone is associated with prolongation of the QT interval (QT interval represents the time for both ventricular depolarisation and repolarisation to occur, and therefore roughly estimates the duration of an average ventricular action potential) of the electrocardiogram, and at higher doses with torsade de pointes (twisting the points),[21] a specific form of ventricular tachycardia. Therefore, caution is required when methadone is prescribed with other drugs that may prolong the QT interval (antipsychotics, tricyclic antidepressants and antiarrhythmics), and in those with pre-existing heart disease. At higher doses, electrocardiogram monitoring is advised.

The unique pharmacological properties of buprenorphine (a partial agonist of the opioid mu receptors – predominant in the brain and spinal cord – with high affinity) leads to the possibility of antagonising the effect of previously administered opioid analgesia or precipitating opiate withdrawal symptoms.

Buprenorphine is partially excreted by the kidney, the majority being excreted in the faeces. Therefore, the dosage does not need to be significantly adjusted in people with renal impairment.[22] Like methadone, buprenorphine is metabolised in the liver, and similarly the activity may be increased, or prolonged, with hepatic impairment. There is evidence that buprenorphine may cause deterioration in liver function in the person with pre-existing liver disease, particularly in overdose, and if tablets are injected.[23,24] Therefore, liver function tests should be checked at the time of initiation, and throughout treatment, the frequency of which may depend on initial results.

SUBUTEX (BUPRENORPHINE), OR SUBOXONE (BUPRENORPHINE AND NALOXONE)?
As with methadone, buprenorphine has the potential to be used recreationally. Sublingual tablets may be crushed into a powder and injected or used intra-nasally, constituting a potentially serious overdose risk.

Suboxone consists of a combination of buprenorphine and the opioid receptor antagonist naloxone. It will produce withdrawal symptoms if not administered sublingually, as prescribed. It should be noted that Suboxone is not currently licensed for use in pregnancy in the UK.

Several other drugs may be effective in the later stages of treatment of persons with substance use issues, particularly to assist with abstinence or to alleviate withdrawal symptoms.

➤ **Naltrexone** is an opioid receptor antagonist ideally used in combination with psychosocial interventions as a treatment for relapse prevention in opiate dependence. It has the propensity to cause severe withdrawal symptoms in the person who is currently taking opiate drugs, and in the individual previously using opiates who has not permitted a sufficient 'wash-out' period. Naltrexone is contraindicated in acute hepatitis or liver failure, and liver function tests should be arranged prior to and after initiation of treatment.

➤ **Acamprosate** is a glutamate receptor antagonist used in chronic alcohol use to maintain abstinence. It is contraindicated in severe liver impairment.

➤ **Lofexidine** is an alpha-2 receptor agonist used in the management of symptoms of opioid withdrawal. The propensity to cause hypotension (and rebound hypertension on withdrawal) and bradycardia requires that extreme caution be taken if prescribed to the individual with severe coronary insufficiency, recent myocardial infarction, bradycardia, hypotension and in pregnancy.

4 To develop an understanding of the social context of the individual

Behaviour, physical and mental health influence, and are influenced by, the environment and social circumstances. Response to treatment and motivation to engage with the substance use service will be affected by issues such as:

➤ employment
➤ housing
➤ interpersonal relationships.

Relationship and financial difficulties can contribute to:
➤ low self-esteem
➤ lack of confidence
➤ further substance use.

However, good family support networks and employment may be protective in terms of assisting abstinence or decreasing the risk of relapse.

5 To identify the main substance of use and to establish degree of dependence

Knowledge of the duration, frequency and means of administration of a substance help to determine the degree of dependence. Tolerance to a substance can be inferred from the amount used, and how the physiological response has changed over time. Therefore, the use of a substance use assessment may be helpful. However, it should be remembered that such 'tools' are an 'aid' and not a replacement for one-to-one interactive assessment.

Questionnaires, such as the Alcohol, Smoking and Substance Use Involvement Screening Test (ASSIST),[25,26] may be used to screen for substance use.

There are other tools, and some might argue that it is a lengthy document for use in the clinical environment. However, the time taken to complete this assessment is dependent on the number of positive responses. ASSIST has been chosen because it:
➤ was developed by the World Health Organization
➤ is based on AUDIT – gold standard alcohol screening tool
➤ screens for the use of:
  — tobacco
  — alcohol
  — cannabis
  — cocaine
  — amphetamine-type stimulants
  — inhalants
  — sedatives/sleeping pills
  — hallucinogens
  — opioids
  — specified others substances.

ASSIST screens for:
➤ substances people have ever used (lifetime use)
➤ substances used in the past three months
➤ problems related to substance use
➤ risk of harm (current or future)
➤ dependence
➤ intravenous (IV) drug use.

The professional completes ASSIST with the individual. ASSIST aids the professional to distinguish between three main groups.

1 Low-risk substance users, or abstainers.
2 Those whose patterns of use put them at risk of problems/who have already developed problems/who are at risk of developing dependence.
3 Those who are dependent on a substance.

ASSIST can:
➤ warn the individual to the risks of developing problems related to the substance of use
➤ provide an opportunity to start a discussion about substance use
➤ identify substance use as a contributing factor to the presenting ill health
➤ be linked to a brief intervention to help individual at high risk to cut down, or stop, the substance(s) of use, and avoid the harmful consequences of the substance use.

How to use ASSIST

An experienced professional can conduct an ASSIST screen, and deliver the integrated brief intervention, in 10–20 minutes. Before screening commences a response card is given to the individual, on which the 'score' is written, and the risk level for each substance used specified. Such intervention provides individual feedback and the professional can offer the appropriate intervention.[25,26]

Physical examination can reveal symptoms and signs of intoxication or withdrawal and injection sites may be visible. Investigations, such as urine testing, provide further evidence of drug use, although blood, saliva and hair testing are also used.

6 To identify other substances of use

Poly drug use (the use of two or more substances) greatly increases the risk of physical health problems and overdose. Often additional drugs are used to potentiate the desirable effects of a preferred drug, or to counteract undesirable side-effects. However, dependence on each substance of use may be present, with such illicit substance use also often being associated with alcohol dependence.[27]

POST-READING EXERCISE 6.1

Time: 10 minutes
List the principal aims of physical health assessment.
Compare your list with the Post-Reading exercise 6.1 answers on p. 78.

CONCLUSION

An eclectic, holistic, person-centred approach to screening and assessment is preferred given that the physical, mental and social aspects of life are often closely interconnected. The process of physical examination begins at the point of entry into the mental health–substance use service and should be regarded as a continuous and dynamic process. All members of the intra- and interdisciplinary teams are involved in the process.

Identifying and treating physical–mental health problems is an integral part of substance use management. Failure to do so hinders treatment in terms of reducing the potential of achieving abstinence and may potentially increase the risk of relapse, if abstinence is achieved. Similarly, an understanding of the social context and its contribution to a person's substance use is imperative.

It is tempting to regard substance use itself as the primary problem. All too often, however, substance use is intrinsically related to psychological distress and associated with social deprivation. Therefore, it is imperative to assess and address the underlying contributory factors to substance use, frequently complicated by physical disease, if we are to assist the person in obtaining abstinence or his/her chosen goal.

REFERENCES

1 Dickey B, Normand SLT, Weiss RD, *et al.* Medical morbidity, mental illness and substance use disorders. *Psychiatr Serv.* 2002; **53**: 862–7.
2 Appleby L, Thomas S, Ferrier N, *et al.* Sudden unexplained death in psychiatric inpatients. *Br J Psychiatry.* 2000; **174**: 405–6.
3 Felker B, Yazel J, Short, D. Mortality and medical co-morbidity among psychiatric patients: a review. *Psychiatr Serv.* 1996; **47**: 1356–63.
4 Hansen V, Arnesen E, Jacobsen BK. Total mortality in people admitted to a psychiatric hospital. *Br J Psychiatry.* 1997; **170**: 186–90.
5 Hippisley-Cox J, Fielding K, Pringle M. Depression as a risk factor for ischaemic heart disease in men: population based case-control study. *BMJ.* 1998; **316**: 1714–19.
6 Goodwin RD, Stein RB. Generalised anxiety disorder and peptic ulcer disease among adults in the United States. *Psychosom Med.* 2002; **64**: 862–6.
7 Lee H. *To Kill a Mockingbird.* London: Mandarin; 1989.
8 Ghuran A, Van Der Wieken LR, Nolan J. Cardiovascular complications of recreational drugs are an important cause of morbidity and mortality. *BMJ.* 2001; **323**: 464–6.
9 Inyang VA, Cooper AJ, Hodgkinson DW. Cocaine induced myocardial infarction. *J Accid Emerg Med.* 1999; **16**: 374–5.
10 Mody CK, Miller BL, McIntyre HB, *et al.* Neurologic complications of cocaine abuse. *Neurology.* 1988; **38**: 1189.
11 Green RM, Kelly KM, Gabrielsen T, *et al.* Multiple cerebral intracerebral haemorrhages after smoking 'crack' cocaine. *Stroke.* 1990; **21**: 957–62.
12 Gossop M, Neto D, Mirjana R, *et al.* Physical health problems among patients seeking treatment for alcohol use disorders: a study in six European cities. *Addict Biol.* 2007; **12**: 190–6.
13 Poschl G, Seitz HK. Alcohol and cancer. *Alcohol Alcohol.* 2004; **39**: 155–65.
14 Boyle MJ, Vella L, Maloney E. Role of drugs and alcohol in patients with head injury. *J R Soc Med.* 1991; **84**: 608–10.
15 Naidoo DP, Bramdev A, Cooper K. Wernicke's encephalopathy and alcohol-related disease. *Postgrad Med J.* 1991; **67**: 978–81.
16 Romero-Gomez M, Boza F, Garcia MS, *et al.* Subclinical hepatic encephalopathy predicts the development of overt hepatic encephalopathy. *Am J Gastroenterol.* 2001; **96**: 2718–23.
17 Baigent MF. Understanding alcohol misuse and comorbid psychiatric disorders. *Curr Opin Psychiatry.* 2005; **18**: 223–8.
18 Simon V, Ho DD, Karim QA. HIV/AIDS epidemiology, pathogenesis, prevention, and treatment. *Lancet.* 2006; **368**: 489–504.

19 Lemon SC, Friedmann PD, Stein MD. The impact of smoking cessation on drug abuse treatment outcome. *Addict Behav.* 2003; **28**: 1323–31.

20 National Institute for Health and Clinical Excellence. *Methadone and Buprenorphine for Managing Opioid Dependence.* TA114. London: National Institute for Health and Clinical Excellence; 2007.

21 Krantz MJ, Lewkowiez L, Hays H, *et al.* Torsade de pointes associated with very-high-dose methadone. *Ann Inter Med.* 2002; **137**: 501–4.

22 Elkader A, Sproule B. Buprenorphine: clinical pharmacokinetics in the treatment of opioid dependence. *Clini Pharmacokinet.* 2005; **44**: 661–80.

23 Berson A, Gervais A, Cazals D, *et al.* Hepatitis after intravenous buprenorphine misuse in heroin addicts. *J Hepatol.* 2001; **34**: 346–50.

24 Herve S, Riachi G, Noblet C, *et al.* Acute hepatitis due to buprenorphine administration. *Euro J Gastroenterol Hepatol.* 2004; **16**: 1033–7.

25 World Health Organization. *The ASSIST project: Alcohol, Smoking and Substance Involvement Screening Test.* Available at: www.who.int/substance_abuse/activities/assist/en/index.html (accessed 14 January 2010).

26 World Health Organization. *ASISST.* Available at: www.who.int/substance_abuse/activities/assist_v3_english.pdf (accessed 14 January 2010).

27 Gossop M, Marsden J, Stewart D. Dual dependence: assessment of dependence upon alcohol and illicit drugs, and the relationship of alcohol dependence among drug misusers to patterns of drinking, illicit drug use and health problems. *Addiction.* 2002; **97**: 168–9.

TO LEARN MORE

Department of Health (UK) and the Developed Administrations. *Drug Misuse and Dependence: UK guidelines on clinical management.* London: Department of Health (England), the Scottish Government, Welsh Assembly Government and Northern Ireland Executive; 2007.

Lishman WA. *Organic Psychiatry: the psychological consequences of cerebral disorder.* 3rd ed. Oxford: Blackwell Science; 1998.

EXERCISE ANSWERS

PRE-READING EXERCISE 6.1 ANSWERS

Starting at the head and working down, below is a list of the physical effects of substance use. This list in not exhaustive and the consequences can consist of more than one physical health problem/complaint.

- Impaired senses – vision, decrease in taste and smell, decrease in the perception of pain
- Altered sense of time and space
- Impaired judgement
- Impaired motor skills
- Hallucinations
- Seizures and blackouts
- Loss of peripheral sensation/tingling
- Dementia
- Wernicke's syndrome
- Psychosis
- Mood and personality changes
- Anxiety
- Brain damage
- Damage to optic nerve
- Cancer of the jaw
- Cancer of the oesophagus
- Cancer of the tongue
- Cancer of the mouth
- High blood pressure
- Irregular heart beat
- Damaged heart muscle
- Cardiovascular event (CVE)
- Collapsed veins
- Irregular heartbeat
- Lung cancer
- Slowed breathing
- Slow heart rate
- Infection of the heart
- Throat, stomach and duodenal ulcers
- Cancer of the stomach
- Cancer of the colon
- Inflammation/irritation of the stomach lining

- Varicose veins of the oesophagus
- Loss of appetite
- Weight loss
- Nausea
- Diarrhoea and vomiting
- Hepatitis B and C
- HIV/AIDS
- Pancreatitis
- Inflamed liver
- Liver cancer
- Oedema
- Increased risk of haemorrhage
- Liver failure, coma and death
- Kidney failure
- Increased micturition
- Foetal alcohol syndrome
- Foetal alcohol effects
- Miscarriage
- Low sperm count
- Reduced fertility
- Impaired sexual performance
- Increased risk of breast cancer
- Irregular menstrual cycle
- Early menopause
- Impaired erectile function
- Weight gain
- Muscle weakness
- Headache
- Migraine
- Vasoconstriction
- Cutaneous and subcutaneous skin and soft tissue abscesses
- Sclerosis
- Thrombosis superficial veins

POST-READING EXERCISE 6.1 ANSWERS

List the principal aims of physical health assessment:
- to identify existing disease (physical and mental)
- to identify those at risk of physical disease and put measures in place to minimise these risks
- consideration and implementation of pharmacological intervention
- to develop an understanding of the social context of the individual
- to identify the main substance of use and to establish degree of dependence
- to identify other substances of use (including alcohol and tobacco).

CHAPTER 7

The experience of illness

Carol Kirby and Oliver D Slevin

> *I think we've a huge problem with alcohol and depression. . . . And they're both often intertwined. People drink to get out of depression, and the more they do that the more depressed they become.*[1]

INTRODUCTION: SETTING THE SCENE

In this chapter we address the issue of 'the experience of the illness' in respect of persons presenting with mental health–substance use. We can and do speak in general terms of common features of such mental health–substance use situations: epidemiological patterns, how 'people' may present, the efficacy of 'treatment' interventions, aftercare and rehabilitation, and so forth. However, the reality of how these forces – mental disorder coupled with substance use – impact upon the individual, what he/she experiences, is at a different level. What is essential is that this is a person, a self, thrown into a world in which he/she lives their daily life.

We all, to differing degrees, struggle with our existence in the world. However, the interaction of mental health–substance use makes the person's struggle not only unique but also exponentially more difficult. In the above opening quotation, the actor Gabriel Byrne (interviewed by his namesake Gay Byrne) expresses from his own experience how these influences may be 'intertwined'. For those of us who as professional and informal carers reach out to such persons, there is a need to achieve insight into this world. Any attempts to genuinely help are doomed to failure if they do not take into account the individual's struggle to cope, to indeed survive. This is in itself sufficient justification for considering this particular form of illness experience. On these arguments, we proceed in this chapter to address the experience of the person with mental health–substance use problems, and how this impacts upon, and is addressed by, the professionals.

STARTING OUT: THE JOURNEY MOTIF

Michael Ondaatje is a Sri Lankan Booker Prize-winning author. His first published book, *Coming through Slaughter*,[2] tells the story of a man called Buddy Bolden who is widely held among some experts to be the first notable jazz musician. Ondaatje weaves together

79

fact and fiction, using fragments from old documents, medical records and dimly recalled accounts, to produce a story that is more powerful than any patchy historical account.

Bolden was a cornet player who lived in the notorious red-light Storyville district of New Orleans at the start of the last century. In this cauldron of human depravity, Bolden worked for a time as a barber, produced a local gossip news-sheet, and played music that was said to be breathtaking in its virtuosity. None of this music survived on record, but those who knew and heard him spoke of Bolden's music as astonishingly creative and spectacular.

Bolden eventually collapsed during a band march with a serious haemorrhage linked to bursting of blood vessels in his neck while playing. Having become increasingly erratic and violent, he was taken to the House of Detention, underwent surgery for his neck injury and was soon afterwards incarcerated in an asylum for the insane. His admission diagnosis was 'Dementia Praecox, Paranoid Type'.

Ondaatje[2] weaves Bolden's story as a journey at different levels. There is a journey through the mainly black neighbourhood of Storyville. Then, Bolden's own journey from the highly charged and tortured life of the extremely creative person, through depression, alcoholism and eventually a decline into what is now labelled schizophrenia. And, finally, in 1907, his journey under police escort through rural Louisiana. Bolden's last journey out, first by train to Baton Rouge, then by horse-drawn cart over 40 miles through the towns of Sunshine and Vachery and finally coming through Slaughter (a small rural township in Louisiana), is to the State Insane Asylum. He never played again. There, a quarter of a century later, Bolden died forgotten and in obscurity.

We cannot of course minimise the experiences of a person who may, for example, be proceeding along the course of a serious and terminal physical illness. The threat to one's very existence is a fearsome encounter. But the experience of someone such as poor Buddy Bolden is a different journey in some ways. We can only imagine that his progression was something akin to the classic Dungeons and Dragons cult game. Here we find someone plunged into the dark dungeons of substance use, while being pursued by the dragons conjured up by a disordered mind. The struggle through these assaults on the self and the journey towards its conclusion almost defy our imagination. But we must try to imagine, we must seek to understand the journey. The journey, in effect, becomes our motif.

The value of the journey motif is indeed even recognised in the modern services for those suffering these conditions. For example, in respect of substance use, current UK healthcare strategy[3] places a greater focus on the journey. It speaks of:

> improving clients journeys through more effective drug treatment and reintegration into local communities (housing, education and employment), [while recognising that] . . . each client's drug treatment journey is different and depends on a range of factors including health status, relationships, nature of the drug problem and the quality of the drug treatment they receive.[3]

Within this journey motif, we have questions in respect of whether substance use places a fragile mind at risk of mental disorder, or whether mental ill health places the individual at increased risk of turning to substance use, such as for self-medication purposes. Certainly, epidemiological studies indicate that over one third of persons with

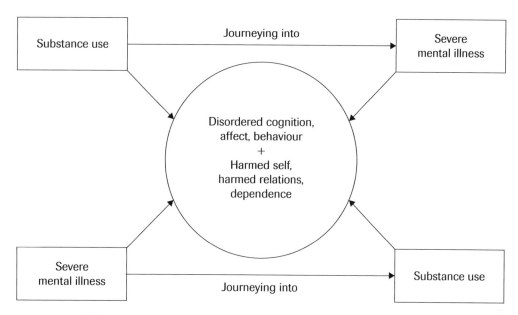

FIGURE 7.1 The mental health–substance use trajectory: different journeys, same outcomes

mental ill health also use substances, while as many as one third to one half of those using substances have mental ill health.[4] Irrespective of which came first, as suggested in Figure 7.1, the burden within the journey includes the ravages of both conditions, each impacting upon the other.

NARRATIVE AS A WINDOW TO EXPERIENCE

The experience of any severe illness is an assault upon the self. Accounts of such disorders by professionals are often expressed in the language of disease that addresses the morbidity, presentation, diagnosis, treatment and outcomes of a malady. But sometimes those who endure such illnesses also give some accounting of what *they* experience. The former accounts – by virtue of their nature (often drawn from medical and epidemiological records) – are characteristically fragmented. They provide partial glimpses of what was experienced, through the intermediary vehicle of often-depersonalised medical nomenclature. The latter accounts – by virtue of *their* nature (in essence being 'storied' accounts) – provide more comprehensive renderings. They are in the nature of a recounted 'lived experience' of what the individual has encountered during an experience that was an ordeal endured.

Considering the two orientations, van Manen[5] speaks of the *gnostic* quest for information and knowledge (the diagnostic seeing through) and the *pathic* quest for a seeing into the self, the suffering being experienced. Elsewhere in this book and in the series we do address the vitally important body of medical and professional knowledge, and the importance of the best available evidence to inform practice. Here, we are concerned with the pathic experiences that narratives can uncover.

It is in the nature of our humanness that we try to derive meaning from that which we experience, that we try to seek order from disorder. The stories here are of course *constructed*. They are searches for meaning, attempts to make sense of and interpret the experience. However, herein lies the danger of seeing meaning where no or different meaning exists, of attributing order to a disordered reality. Life, as the old saying goes, is not like that! This quest for meaning is Odyssean in so far as it attempts to present a story that has a beginning, a progression through illness, and an end that represents some point of closure or arrival – whether it is the end of a life or some form of emancipation or arrival once again into the light. From such narratives we gain insights, it is true. But we must also subject them to our critical interpretive gaze: they are, after all, constructions. This is not necessarily a bad thing. From such hermeneutic scrutiny, the reader/listener is gifted with the opportunity to extend the circle of interpretation. Horizons fuse, as the teller's unfolding story horizon comes together with the interpreting horizon of the listener, into something that can reasonably be claimed a deepening of understanding.

Stories are *recounted*. They are 'tellings' that have as their objective the conveying to another of an experience. The teller has a purpose: he/she wishes to relate the experience. There is a need for whatever reasons to let the other who will listen know. The teller is saying: this is what happened to me; this is what it was like; this is what it means to be suffering in this way. The key term here is the word 'relate'. At a superficial level we can see this as meaning to speak out or to tell. But at a deeper level there is a reaching out to the 'other', an attempt to really convey the experience in its fullest sense. It is in this relationship between self and other that the teller proceeds to make sense of this journey through illness. The *other* becomes in a sense *self*, a mirror, through which each of us gains a reflection of our own life. And for the listener, who must become this other, there is a demand to respond to the story.

This is always a challenge, insofar as it calls the listener to attempt to enter into the life of this self, this person experiencing an illness. For a listener who is in an optimal state of health and well-being, who perhaps has never been seriously ill, this is particularly difficult. It has been suggested that for a person who has never themselves been ill, who has not experienced the particular illness in question, the attempt to reach real insight into the experience is illusive. In this respect, the literature around the concept of *the wounded healer* is informative.[6–11] This derives from the ancient Greek myth of Chiron. The centaur Chiron was said to have been accidentally wounded in the knee by a poisoned arrow, from which healing was not possible. Chiron suffered great pain for the remainder of his life. He retired to a cave to attempt the futile task of healing himself. However, through his search for healing and his awareness of pain he developed the wisdom and insight to become a great healer for others, though never for himself. A theme in the Chiron myth is that through suffering ourselves we become more sympathetic to the pain of others, and more able to respond to their need for healing.

Listening, then, becomes just as important as the telling. We always 'tell' to the 'listener', even if this is oneself. Unfortunately, in our modern-day fast technological world, listening is not always given to us. Yet, it is this receptiveness to the voice of the other that is the gateway to understanding what that other is experiencing. Of this, Illich said:

First among the classification of the silences is the silence of the pure listener, of womanly passivity; the silence through which the message of the other becomes 'he in us', the silence of deep interest. It is threatened by another silence – the silence of indifference, the silence of disinterest which assumes there is nothing I want or can receive through the communication of the other.[12]

It is this 'deep interest' in the other that opens up the world of the sufferer. This is reinforced by the call of Paul Solomon:[13]

If I want to know what you're thinking right now, all I have to do is care more about what you're thinking than what I'm thinking. . . . As soon as I care more about what you're thinking than what I'm thinking I will give up my thoughts and I will absorb yours, and I will understand you.[13]

When we *do* care about what the other tells, when that other does become 'he in us', we in effect address the *pathic*.[5] We embrace the person's *pathos* or experience: and this we call *empathy*. We know, to as great an extent as is possible, what that other is thinking, feeling, experiencing.[14,15]

REFLECTIVE PRACTICE EXERCISE 7.1   Willing to listen

Time: 20 minutes

In her book *Agnes's Jacket*, the psychologist Gail Hornstein stated:

When I began studying psychology seriously in graduate school, I was startled to learn that psychotic patients were supposed to be too 'narcissistic' and 'unrelational' to allow others into their inner worlds. The people I had gotten to know in the dozens of patient narratives I had read by then didn't seem anything like the cases in textbooks. My professors were puzzled and vaguely suspicious of my interests in madness literature . . . so I learned not to talk about these . . .[16]

Reflect upon the assertion that concerned Hornstein that psychotic patients are 'unrelational'.

- Do you agree with this assertion?
- Even if it is agreed that relating to such individuals is difficult, how do you think we can gain some insight into what they are experiencing?
- Do we have to look for different terms of engagement for such persons?

TERMS OF ENGAGEMENT: TOWARDS ACTIVE LISTENING

There is a need to consider the role of the listener in moving towards a fuller understanding of the illness experience. It cannot be assumed that a true listening orientation exists. Indeed, mental health–substance use services do not always provide a listening space. There are certainly well documented analyses that highlight a disease-orientated dominant discourse and the medicalisation of social problems as illness.[16-19] At worst, such orientations can move too rapidly from obtaining objectified, scientific informa-tion to medical (pharmaceutical and other) responses to symptom control. Assuming this hurdle can be overcome, a listening receptivity to the other can be sought. However, the capacity to achieve deep empathy is dependent on moving beyond *passive listening* to a more *active listening* mode. This requires the establishment of a close and trust-ing relationship, within which, through two-way dialogue and feedback over time, the listener's understanding of the other is increasingly enhanced.[20,21]

In mental health–substance use problems the challenge is one of gaining access to and understanding fractured lives when the very window to that understanding, the accounts of sufferers, is also fractured and broken. Those who use substances often live covert and secret lives, outside of the law and in private torment, unseen by others unless sometimes those of their own kind; their stories are reluctant and guarded, and often secret. Those suffering a psychotic illness are often cut off from reality, plagued by delusions and fears, with the cognitive capacity to make sense of and express their deranged world compromised; their stories are at best distorted and often incompre-hensible. We might view this in terms of separate stories that are already difficult being made more difficult by becoming one complex story, as suggested in Figure 7.2. The problem is accentuated when the sufferer is confronted by a confusing array of services, often speaking in different or even opposing voices, and not always interested in that individual's personal story.

REFLECTIVE PRACTICE EXERCISE 7.2 Windows on experience – joining up paradigms

---

Time: 20 minutes

It is sometimes suggested that in the course of previous decades mental health–substance use services have developed as two entirely separate orientations, each with their different underlying values and philosophies, and each operating within markedly different paradigms or worldviews.

On such an argument, it is suggested that the mental health services operate within a medical-scientific paradigm that emphasises objectification of problems, and a case-orientated approach to diagnosing and treating disease. Conversely, it is suggested that substance use services operate within a social-psychological-human science paradigm that emphasises the importance of self within context and a person-orientated approach to resolving problems of adjustment and living.

It is further suggested that each service has developed within entirely different care systems, with substance use services lacking insight into mental health problems, and mental health services lacking insight into substance use problems.

- Reflect upon the arguments for justifying the above assertions.
- Consider what implications such circumstances (separate and opposing paradigms) may have for the individual with mental health–substance use problems.
- Does the paradigm (context) affect the story?
- Reflect upon the possibility of a third/new/different paradigm that may be more appropriate for responding to the needs of the individual with mental health–substance use problems.
- Consider actual examples of new ways of working in such circumstances.
- Consider in particular coordinated, multidisciplinary and integrated care orientations.

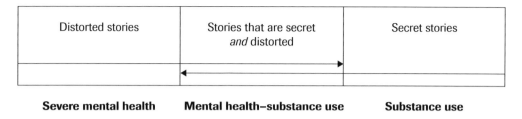

Distorted stories	Stories that are secret *and* distorted	Secret stories

Severe mental health   **Mental health–substance use**   **Substance use**

FIGURE 7.2 The mental health–substance use experience: worst of both worlds

POINTS ALONG THE WAY

We might advance our quest for understanding by drawing upon our knowledge of what are termed stages in the illness journey. Such signposting has been suggested by a number of sources. The most commonly cited approach among so-called *stage models* of serious illness, bereavement and death is that originally proposed by Kubler-Ross,[22] but later applied to wider circumstances such as traumatic life events.[23] Kubler-Ross suggested the following five stages.

1   **Denial**: this defence mechanism of refusing to accept the illness (or prospect of dying) is usually only a temporary defence for the individual.
2   **Anger**: this is an aggressive response to the situation, often reflected in a 'why me' attitude.
3   **Bargaining**: there is some degree of coming to terms with the situation, often accompanied by attempts to contain or through negotiation and rationalisation establish a cessation or delay in the progression towards death, and perhaps also still a degree of hope in reversal of the process.
4   **Depression**: a realisation that one is not going to have a stay or reversal, that all there is left is a proceeding towards demise, accompanied often by distress, mood depression and withdrawal.
5   **Acceptance**: the coming to terms with one's destiny as determined by the disease's course, an acceptance of the inevitable destiny.[22]

Adopting a similar stage model, though drawing upon the more existential idea of a journey through terminal illness, a nine-stage approach[11] can be suggested that is expressed in terms of processes in a journey, not necessarily in an orderly sequence but in a more convoluted way, and including the following elements.

1   **Awareness**: a realisation that all is not well, that things are different. That in one's mind or body one is not functioning as before: there is an awareness that something is wrong, an experiencing of pain, or distress, or dysfunction.
2   **Being and non-being**: a confrontation with mortality, the prospect of being sick, or even dying. This may reach its highest level, often accompanied by severe angst (survival anxiety), when a diagnosis is made and bad news is conveyed. There is an acute consciousness of one's being and a confronting of the possibility of non-being. The philosopher Heidegger[24] viewed this in terms of the capacity within each person for authentic or inauthentic being. For the person, healthy or well, there is a choice of authentically confronting one's existence and inevitable non-existence, or inauthentically choosing to avoid the angst of this acute awareness. In the case of

the severely ill person, Young recognises inauthentic being as a tranquillising 'flight from death'.[25]

3 **Separation, confronting mortality alone**: one enters the world of being a sick person. This is a form of status passage whereby the person has become different, set apart, by virtue of this becoming. Using more mechanistic terminology, we might view this as adopting what has become termed a sick role.[26] Here, the individual relinquishes personal freedom and becomes a compliant follower of the prescriptions of treatment: others become responsible as old roles are (permanently or temporarily) relinquished. At an existential level, there is the sense of now being set apart, as the afflicted one. And with this, the important realisation that at one level each must face his/her destiny alone.

4 **The lived experience of suffering**: there may be physical incapacity. There may be emotional distress or (in the case of mental or neurological illness) cognitive disturbance. There may be pain (mild or extreme) of a physical and/or emotional quality. While such pain may be ameliorated or relieved through therapeutic intervention, one is now enduring an assault upon the self, perhaps beyond anything the person might previously have imagined. This suffering and enduring becomes central to one's existence.

5 **Avoiding reality and seeking meaning**: as one proceeds through these experiences, there are varying degrees of attempts to avoid/deny the illness. There is also an attempt to understand what is happening, to seek meaning. In respect of terminal illness,[27] some incurably ill individuals do seek to understand and come to terms with the situation, while others may continue, perhaps for the duration of the illness, to adopt a constant position of denial.

6 **Living life as it is given, facing illness and death as it approaches**: eventually, each person arrives at some form of acceptance, or (as suggested above) proceeds in a state of *rejection* or denial that indeed may never be resolved. Having endured a status passage, a mode of living is embarked upon.

7 **Appraising the past**: in some instances, particularly where individuals in a terminal illness do confront the prospect of an end, there is an appraisal of past life. This can range from a desire to put things in order or to reach closure on unfinished business, to high degrees of distress and regret regarding past failures. Indeed, the degree of distress can lead to such high levels of agitation that it even impacts upon the effectiveness of pain relief interventions.[27]

8 **Living now**: to whatever degree a person has proceeded through processes of awareness or denial, acceptance or rejection, an authentic and searching quest for meaning or an inauthentic choice to live in denial, each is a living being that for the present continues to live, in some way. This 'living now' may take the form of simply surviving within the cloak of palliative care or day-to-day routine. It may involve a determination to achieve something held dear, or simply to be there for dependent others for as long as possible. In fact, this will be different for each individual.

9 **Facing the end**: the course of a serious disorder, particularly a terminal physical disease, presents the prospect of death. This is in effect a confrontation with the unknown. The ravages of a diseased body and mind, the cultural context and belief systems that are part of the person's inner being, how the person progressed through the illness and the meaning they attributed to this journey, all come together to

influence the approach to and through the dying process. For some, the final relief from pain is welcomed. Others, whose spirituality is anchored in religious beliefs, anticipate a life hereafter.[7] For yet others, there is a consuming fear and dread. Each approaches this end point in his/her own way; and, in the final moments, each arrives there alone.[11]

The problem with such 'stage models' is that the empirical support of their relevance in real-life situations is rather elusive. This is indeed strongly argued by some[28,29] who suggests that while there *is* a dearth of empirical evidence on such models, the most convincing evidence is that people do not proceed through such discrete stages within given time frames. Some people proceed through grieving processes quickly; others may remain in denial for the remainder of their lives. Conversely, some evidence supporting the stage model in respect of persons grieving natural death bereavements has been identified.[30] The argument for stage models often draws upon strong anecdotal accounts, and the acceptance of stage models by notable authorities such as palliative care specialists and medical school educators. In fairness, in her later writing and teaching Kubler-Ross recognised that her model was a broad guide.[22,23] Similarly Slevin,[11] presented the idea that in the experience of a serious illness the processes are by definition convoluted rather than orderly and sequential.

Interestingly, and perhaps supporting the validity of the stage models perspective, experience in mental health tends to mirror that in respect of serious physical illness and death and bereavement. A literature review encompassing research, consumer accounts, theoretical literature and personal accounts[31] identified clear patterns of a staged journey through schizophrenia and other serious mental illness. Moving from an initial point of distress (variously described as a moratorium, crisis, being overwhelmed), through struggling to come to terms and establish meaning while living with the disability, to a rebuilding or restructuring of one's self, and finally some degree of growth and living beyond the disability or through coping with the disability. Similarly, in work extending over more than 15 years it was found that those who suffer serious mental illness characterised by 'hearing voices' proceed through a phase of being 'startled' (anxious and overwhelmed), though a phase of 'organisation' (seeking understanding and meaning) to a phase of 'stabilisation' (recovery of potential and capacities).[32-4]

Processes, such as those outlined in stage models, may help us understand the experiences of illness as they unfold in stories and dialogue about these stories. However, we cannot assume a common roadmap: each person's journey is different, and so too is each story. But we can recognise patterns, as and when they arise, that help us interpret the experience. Beyond that, the listener-helper can know from such pointers:

➤ when to respond supportively to distress, confusion and anxiety
➤ when to engage in a quest for understanding and meaning
➤ when to support the reconstruction of a life.

REFLECTIVE PRACTICE EXERCISE 7.3 Larry David smokes weed

Time: 20 minutes
Access this source by searching for 'Larry David smokes weed' or 'Larry David gets stoned' on the website www.youtube.com.

This is a YouTube video. In this comedy sketch (which may not be entirely tasteful) the well-known comedian has obtained marijuana to help his father's glaucoma. Being himself cajoled into taking the substance he has an unpleasant experience. While the sketch has comic aspects there is also a serious side: an extreme reaction to substance use. The hallucinatory experiences represented in the sketch are akin to those documented in substance use literature, and indeed are not dissimilar to those in serious mental illnesses.

- Open and view the video.
- Reflect on how Larry is apparently distressed by the experience.
- Reflect on how individuals may be plagued by such experiences (hearing voices) day in and day out.

You will note that while the character is being berated by the voice in a threatening fashion, the issues (diet, lifestyle, relationships, etc.), may very well be matters that concern the Larry character himself. Assuming his distress is at least for a time abated:

- How might you discuss with him what was happening here, what the voice was saying?

EXPERIENCING MENTAL HEALTH–SUBSTANCE USE: THE CASE FOR ASSISTED STORYTELLING

At this point it is useful to summarise the position thus far, as follows.

1 **Reaching out**: we argue that if we are to reach out, to help those with a mental health–substance use problem, we need to bring together a range of suitable expertise and support (ideally, intra- and interdisciplinary), but that *the individual's perspective is core*. Our justification for addressing the illness experience is the enhancement of our capacity to respond.

2 **Person-centred approach**: a corollary to this orientation is the necessity of a *person-centred approach* to care. In the confluence of severe mental illness and substance use, it is important to recognise that each instance will be unique to a significant extent. We cannot expect detailed protocols or standardised guidelines that will carry validity or indeed relate reliably to each and every case. We indeed must move from a case to a person orientation, based upon a caring and trusting relationship particularly when the person's experience is one of mistrust of self and of other.

3 **The journey orientation**: we have also argued for a *journey motif*, suggesting that we can achieve insight by exploring the individual's progression through illness. This orientation maintains focus upon the individual's experience.

4 **Listening**: the window to this experience is *the story as narrated by the individual* and as heard by we who listen. The willingness to listen is of vital importance, and extends from a passive yet attentive listening to a narrative, to a more active and reflective listening through dialogue.

5 **Perceiving patterns**: we can turn to aids such as *stage models of illness* that provide pointers to what we might listen for. While each ill person's experience, and thus story, is unique there are nevertheless patterns of processes and responses that when recognised may illuminate and increase our understanding of what is being experienced.

6 **Adopting a reflexive orientation**: the circumstances surrounding mental health–substance use are complex. The social responses, in terms of stigma and social exclusion, and different worldviews underpinning service provisions are complex. The experiencing of an illness that has both mental illness and substance use characteristics is also complex. Within such complexity, the stories emerging are frequently chaotic. We must constantly adopt a *reflexive approach* that seeks patterns and meanings that are themselves constantly in flux.

7 **Procuring an authentic story**: as a consequence, what often emerges from such circumstances may be *stories that are distorted and secret*. Where the *storyteller* is cognitively incapacitated through mental illness, the story may be so distorted as to challenge interpretation and understanding. Where substance use is often kept private and hidden, indeed covert and secret (often for legal and social reasons), the procuring of a true and authentic story is a challenge, requiring the establishment of trust and mutual regard.

When we consider the lived experience of someone coping with mental ill health and substance use problems simultaneously, we are (as indicated at item 6 above) confronted with an additional challenge. Severe mental illness and substance use share one significant characteristic: both are by definition stigmatising, conveying moral stain. Those labelled as seriously mentally ill or substance users are sometimes construed as folk devils[35] – perceived as dangerous and unpredictable (mentally ill), or socially degenerate and criminal (substance use). As such, the burden is increased as social exclusion and even overt discrimination becomes an even more significant part of the illness experience. This experience – often including being distressed and disturbed, substance dependent, excluded and alone, demonised – necessitates from carers exceptional capacities for humanity, insight and understanding.

Faced with such circumstances, and a person both seriously ill and marginalised, it is tempting to abort all attempts at making sense of what the ill person is experiencing. Confronted by distrust and irrationality, it may seem the way forward is impossible. We must nevertheless seek what understanding and insight we can derive from this situation. This is accommodated by returning to the interpretive-hermeneutic orientation identified earlier. That is, the suggestion that for any story (no matter how apparently irrational or reluctantly shared) there is a teller and a listener. In this sense, the story becomes a co-creation wherein the storyteller's attempt to establish and convey meaning is responded to by the listener's attempt to gain understanding and insight. There is of course an argument that active participation by the listener would take away from the authenticity of the story. It is, after all, someone else's story.

This might be considered in terms of the idea of an *emic* and *etic* voice, used within anthropology.[36] The *emic* voice is that of the native, that of the insider within a culture. It is an insider's voice contextualised within that culture, understandable to those in that culture and within that context. The *etic* voice is that of the outsider, and thus is an attempt to interpret and understand from the point of view of that outsider's cultural perspective. Herein lies the risk of applying interpretations that, while appropriate in a different setting, have little or no currency in the one being observed. Therefore, it is important in the process of co-creating the story that the listener focuses primarily on the insider's voice, on the *emic* view, and collaborates in the clarifying and expression of that story.

Therefore, it is not producing a *joint* story, but still, in the final analysis, a production of the experiencing person's story. In this sense, we might view it as *assisted storytelling*. This is justified on the argument that for the individual with mental health–substance use concerns and dilemmas, one facet of their illness is an incapacity or reduced capacity to rationally construct a story. It is important to recognise that this is not necessarily the same as constructing a *rational* story. Indeed, the story insofar as it is an account of what the individual experiences it is more likely to be a story of a fractured life wherein the quest to make sense of a confused existence is as distressing for the individual as confusing for the listener, and where the turning to non-prescription substances use may indeed be an attempt to escape this situation.

The idea of utilising an assisted storytelling perspective has some merit. Kirby extends the call to listening referred to above by pointing to the necessity of interpreting the experience and meaning of illness for each person as a 'body-mind-spirit' entity. She states:

> Individual suffering is in every way unique. Access to the suffering and loss that a person is experiencing is inalienably theirs to give. It is an arrogance, intended or not, to believe that we know anything of another's experience other than through their telling. . . . Each person is living and experiencing their unfolding life and its meaning, daily finding and renewing meaning. It is not possible to confer meaning upon another person's life. What is possible and vital . . . is the assistance of the person to find meaning in what they are going through.[37]

In an approach in line with such an orientation, Cooper and Cooper[38] demonstrate how, drawing from case information and individuals accounts, important themes in a person's journey through illness (in this instance, within palliative care) can be identified.

Drawing on such insights we might now extend our earlier seven summary points, as follows:

1 **Assisted storytelling**: recognising the likelihood of some incapacity for the individual experiencing mental health–substance use problems to express their experiences (by virtue of their illness incapacity *and* the complex nature of their circumstances), there is merit in adopting an *assisted storytelling perspective* that allows the listener to participate in co-creating the individual's story.

2 **Primacy of the *emic* voice**: in adopting the latter perspective, it is vitally important to focus upon the *emic* voice of the teller. There are *etic* voices here that include those from the considerable experience of the intra- and interdisciplinary mental health–substance use care team. But these must be harnessed to respecting the primacy of the individual's account, conferring only the meaning (or lack of meaning) that that person's articulation of the experience supports. There are of course various healthcare issues of concern here: the stabilisation of mental health, coping with substance use, addressing nutrition and physical health, and so forth. However, until the *person-centred experience* is articulated, there can be no *person-centred planning* of the journey on to recovery.

It is suggested that these summarised points from our discussion can also serve as a guide to not only uncovering the individual's experience but also responding positively to that account.

REFLECTIVE PRACTICE EXERCISE 7.4 The individual experience

Time: 20 minutes

In the latter section of the chapter we have suggested a number of points that may help in not only exploring the experience of a person with a mental health–substance use problem but, also, how we might respond to these appropriately.

   If you have any experience of contact with or working with a person with a mental health–substance use problem, consider how the points in the latter section may have helped in such situations. If you wish to extend upon these reflections, the two Internet videos, and Internet source on 'hearing voices', below may provide further examples.

   A mental health–substance use dramatisation video: www.inexcess.tv/?p=5982&v=1

   A substance user's story on video: www.inexcess.tv/?p=6039&paged=2&v=1

   A site that explores experiences of those hearing voices: www.intervoiceonline.org/

- Reflect upon how the individual with a substance use problem, a serious mental illness, or indeed both, attempts to make sense of his/her experiences.
- Reflect on whether these stories might make helpers' responses more effective.

CONCLUSION

In this chapter we have attempted to explore the experience of illness for the person with mental health–substance use problems. We draw attention to the difficult task that faced us and, more importantly, faces those with mental health–substance use problems, and the professional. That is, the challenge of accessing experiences where a feature of the circumstances is the inaccessibility and sometimes incomprehensibility of those very experiences. We hope that in sharing our views we have made some contribution to recognition of the difficulties faced. Further to that, the nine summary points presented in the latter section of this chapter are proposed as helpful pointers in working towards an assisted storytelling approach.

   We conclude by a brief reflection on the value of the story, or more specifically, the value of exploring the lived experience of the individual with mental health–substance use problems. Those who study the use of narrative in the human sciences recognise that the telling of a story always has some function. It can be suggested that illness stories can be of chaos, quest and restitution.[6] It is certainly the case that, in the darkest hours, those experiencing a serious mental illness *and* a substance use problem are living through a chaos narrative. An important aspect of their recovery will be their quest for meaning and, eventually, a restored life. In this, there may indeed be an argument for the listener-carer accompanying the person on this journey. It then becomes a journey, a story, for all of us. We might all be rich from the journey.[39]

> . . . off into the world that waits
> between tomorrow and today,

to seek our fortunes and our fates, driven by this yearning,
to be rich from the journey,
rich from the journey.[38]

REFERENCES

1 Byrne G. Interviewed by Byrne G. In: *The Meaning of Life with Gay Byrne.* RTE One; Sunday, 17 January 2010.
2 Ondaatje M. *Coming Through Slaughter.* Toronto, ON: Anansi Press; 1973.
3 National Treatment Agency for Substance Misuse. *Models of Care for Treatment of Adult Drug Users: 2006 update.* London: National Treatment Agency for Substance Misuse; 2006.
4 Marshall J. Dual diagnosis: co-morbidity of severe mental illness and substance misuse. *J Forens Psychiatry Psychol.* 1998; **9**: 9–15.
5 van Manen M. Phenomenology of practice. *Phenomenol Pract.* 2007; **1**: 11–30.
6 Frank A. *The Wounded Storyteller: body, illness and ethics.* Chicago, IL: University of Chicago Press; 1995.
7 Slevin O. Spirituality and nursing. In Basford L, Slevin O, editors. *Theory and Practice of Nursing: an integrated approach to caring practice.* 2nd ed. Cheltenham: Nelson Thornes; 2003.
8 Nouwen H. *The Wounded Healer.* London: Darton, Longman and Todd; 1997.
9 Nouwen H. *Reaching Out.* London: Fount; 1998.
10 Kirby C. Commitment to care. In: Basford L, Slevin O, editors. *Theory and Practice of Nursing: an integrated approach to caring practice.* 2nd ed. Cheltenham: Nelson Thornes; 2003.
11 Slevin O. The experience of illness. In: Cooper J, editor. *Stepping into Palliative Care 1: relationships and responses.* 2nd ed. Oxford: Radcliffe Publishing; 2006.
12 Illich I. *Celebration of Awareness.* Harmondsworth: Penguin; 1973.
13 Solomon P. Paul Solomon speaks on spiritual roots and the journey to wholeness. *Human Potential Magazine.* 1991; **16**: 28–32.
14 Rogers C. The necessary and sufficient conditions of therapeutic personality change. *J Consult Psychol.* 1957; **21**: 95–103.
15 Berger D. *Clinical Empathy.* Northvale, NJ: Jason Aronson, Inc; 1987.
16 Hornstein G. *Agnes's Jacket: a psychologist's search for the meaning of madness.* New York, NY: Rodale Press; 2009. p. 15.
17 Szasz T. *The Myth of Mental Illness.* London: Paladin; 1962.
18 Foucault M. *The Birth of the Clinic.* London: Tavistock; 1976.
19 Illich I. *Limits to Medicine – Medical Nemesis: the expropriation of health.* Harmondsworth: Pelican; 1977.
20 Marangoni C, Garcia S, Ickes W, *et al.* Empathic accuracy in a clinically relevant setting. *J Pers Soc Psychol.* 1995; **18**: 854–69.
21 Ickes W, editor. *Empathic Accuracy.* New York, NY: Guilford Press; 1997.
22 Kubler-Ross E. *On Death and Dying.* London: Tavistock; 1969.
23 Kubler-Ross E, Kessler D. *On Grief and Grieving: finding the meaning of grief through the five stages of loss.* London: Simon & Schuster Ltd; 2005.
24 Heidegger M. *Being and Time.* Oxford: Basil Blackwell; 1962.
25 Young J. Death and authenticity. In: Malpas J, Solomon R, editors. *Death and Philosophy.* New York, NY: Routledge; 1998.
26 Parsons T. *The Social System.* New York, NY: Free Press; 1951.
27 Kearney M. *Mortally Wounded: stories of soul pain, death and healing.* Dublin: Marino Books; 1996.

28 Wortman C, Silver R. The myths of coping with loss. *J Consult Clin Psychol.* 1989; **7**: 349–57.

29 Bonanno G. *The Other Side of Sadness.* New York, NY: Basic Books; 2009.

30 Maciejewski P, Zhang B, Block S, *et al.* An empirical examination of the stage theory of grief. *JAMA.* 2007; **297**: 716–23.

31 Andresen R, Oades L, Caputi P. The experience of recovery from schizophrenia: towards an empirically validated stage model. *Austr N Z J Psychiatry.* 2003; **37**: 586–94.

32 Romme M, Escher S. *Accepting Voices.* London: MIND; 1993.

33 Romme M, Escher S. *Making Sense of Voices.* London: MIND; 2000.

34 Romme M, Escher S, Dillon J, *et al. Living with Voices: 50 stories of recovery.* Ross-on-Wye: PCCS Books; 2009.

35 Cohen S. *Folk Devils and Moral Panics (30th Anniversary Edition).* London: Paladin; 2002.

36 Geertz C. *Local Knowledge.* New York, NY: Basic Books; 1983. p. 85.

37 Kirby C. The therapeutic relationship. In: Cooper J, editor. *Stepping into Palliative Care 1: relationships and responses.* 2nd ed. Oxford: Radcliffe Publishing; 2006.

38 Cooper J, Cooper DB. Hope and coping strategies. In: Cooper J, editor. *Stepping into Palliative Care 1: relationships and responses.* 2nd ed. Oxford: Radcliffe Publishing; 2006.

39 Rhodes K. Rich from the journey. In: Rhodes K. *Rich from the Journey.* Austin, TX: Sunbird Records (CD Recording); 2000.

TO LEARN MORE

Frank A. *The Wounded Storyteller: body, illness and ethics.* Chicago, IL: University of Chicago Press; 1995.

Kirby C. Commitment to care. In: Basford L, Slevin O, editors. *Theory and Practice of Nursing: an integrated approach to caring practice.* 2nd ed. Cheltenham: Nelson Thornes; 2003.

Nouwen H. *The Wounded Healer.* London: Darton, Longman and Todd; 1997.

Nouwen H. *Reaching Out.* London: Fount; 1998.

Saunders C. Foreword. In: Kearney M. *Mortally Wounded: stories of soul pain, death and healing.* Dublin: Marino Books; 1996.

Slevin O. Spirituality and nursing. In: Basford L, Slevin O, editors. *Theory and Practice of Nursing: an integrated approach to caring practice.* 2nd ed. Cheltenham: Nelson Thornes; 2003.

Slevin O. The experience of illness. In: Cooper J, editor. *Stepping into Palliative Care 1: relationships and responses.* 2nd ed. Oxford: Radcliffe Publishing; 2006.

CHAPTER 8

The psychological impact of serious illness

Alyna Turner and Amanda L Baker

INTRODUCTION

Mental health–substance use problems can take a variety of forms. Mental health problems may range from mild symptoms of depression or anxiety to severe mental disorders, which may include severe depression or anxiety, such as post-traumatic stress disorder, and psychoses, such as schizophrenia and bipolar affective disorder.

Psychoactive substance use can also be seen on a continuum. It may be defined as 'problematic' if the use of a legal drug exceeds national health guidelines. However, while problematic use may place a person at risk for future health problems, it may not be associated with any immediately obvious discernible negative psychological or functional difficulties. At the other end of the spectrum, use of a substance may become the primary focus of a person's day-to-day life, impacting on their social environment, role and identity, and physical and mental health.

Although media coverage of substance use tends to emphasise the dangers of illicit drugs, virtually any psychoactive substance can be used. Legal substances (tobacco and alcohol) are associated with the greatest burden of illness and use of such substances is often viewed as normal and encouraged in many societies. Medically supported or controlled substances, such as benzodiazepines for anxiety treatment, opiates for pain relief, or amphetamines for attention deficit hyperactivity disorder, may be prescribed but can be used by others, or diverted for supply to other people. Substances designed for use in everyday life, such as glue, paint or petrol, are psychoactive and can be used. Illicit substances, such as cannabis, cocaine, heroin, ecstasy, amphetamines, opiates and so on, are used internationally, with certain substances being more prevalent in some countries than others, largely depending on availability (supply). Substance use may be occasional or experimental, instrumental (e.g. amphetamines used by truck drivers), infrequent and heavy (e.g. weekend binge drinking) or regular (hazardous, harmful or dependent).

This chapter focuses on the impact of more severe conditions to include regular substance use (that impacts negatively on an individual's day-to-day life) in the context of mental health problems (that are pervasive and not transitory reactions to difficult life situations). Thus the focus is on mental health conditions that would generally meet diagnostic criteria for moderate to severe depression, anxiety or for psychosis and on coexisting substance use.

IMPACT OF MENTAL HEALTH–SUBSTANCE USE

Mental health or substance use problems individually bring their own set of difficulties, which have been described comprehensively. However, mental health–substance use problems bring with them additional unique challenges for the person and the treating professional. Mental health–substance use problems are very common, especially in treatment settings.[1,2] Once the two conditions coexist, this can worsen the course of both conditions and can compromise the treatment response compared to either disorder alone.[3] Taking an example of a person with a severe mental disorder, like schizophrenia, such a person may have lower employment and earning capacity, leading them to live in poorer housing (which may result in greater access to substances). This person would have reduced ability and opportunity to develop social connections except for those in a similar deprived situation, including substance users. In addition, this individual might experience cognitive dysfunctions that might be associated with choices that may result in victimisation and substance use. Substance use may then worsen their psychiatric symptoms, contribute to relapse, and increase the likelihood of social, family, economic, safety and legal difficulties. Conversely, in people with substance use problems, coexisting mental health problems may lead to worse health, social and legal outcomes.

These social, economic and legal difficulties will impact on, and be affected by, the person's view of their behaviour, themselves and the world. Their family and friends will also be unavoidably involved, either through remaining in the situation to provide support, or by choosing to opt out. The impact of mental health–substance use problems on the individual and family, with regard to their personal and psychological experiences, is discussed below.

PART 1: LIVING IN A MENTAL HEALTH–SUBSTANCE USE WORLD

The individual is not isolated, but part of a family, culture and multiple systems (for example, legal, medical and government). All of these factors will impact on their experience of living with mental health–substance use problems.

Substance use itself is not necessarily a problem. As stated above, the use of some psychoactive substances, particularly alcohol, may be encouraged and seen as a positive social behaviour in particular situations. The degree of use seen as acceptable will vary according to social, cultural and religious norms. Therefore, the judgement placed on the person will be situation specific. Having a high alcohol tolerance is admired in particular groups. However, while heavy use may be condoned at the pub or at a party, being intoxicated on the street in the middle of the day would generally result in a different response.

Generational and subcultural influences will also play a role. Smoking tobacco and drinking alcohol were part of the Oldest and Lucky Generations culture; the 'hippy' era encompassing the teenage years of the Baby Boomers was linked in to cannabis and hallucinogenic substance use; while 'party drugs' like ecstasy, and stronger cannabis choices, have become linked to Generation X and Y's socialisation.

While by definition mental disorders are always problematic for the individual, how the person reacts to and expresses their distress, their choice to inform others, and the response of others to that person, are all susceptible to these same influences. A 'traditional older male' may be surprised by, and find his self-concept essentially undermined by, a diagnosis of depression, while a young female whose peer group members have similar diagnoses may be relatively accepting of her own diagnosis.

Social, cultural, religious and generational influences play a role in the person's experience of mental health problems, their substance choice, their perception of their substance use and the experience of stigma. This will also impact on the individual's and family's beliefs around whether the conditions are a problem or not, and whether or not assistance should be sought.

Stigma and mental health–substance use problems

Stigma is the process of marginalisation and ostracism, rejection or disapproval of a particular group of people who are perceived as different in some way compared to others. People with mental health–substance use problems are often seen as inherently different, and therefore engender misunderstanding, prejudice, confusion and fear in the general public. The experience of this ostracism is potentially worse for the person and their loved ones than the illnesses themselves.

Stigma and society

People with severe mental disorders, particularly psychosis, are often viewed with fear and as potentially violent, while people with depression may be seen as negative, morose and weak willed. Substance users may be seen as unpredictable, out of control and potentially violent. Degree of stigma of 18 different situations was evaluated across 14 countries, with drug addiction identified as the most stigmatised, with alcoholism the fourth, and chronic mental disorder the eighth.[4]

The existence of mental health–substance use problems alone does not necessarily mean that stigma will be encountered. For example, an executive being treated with an antidepressant who has a regular, high alcohol intake as expected in his/her job role, may face less stigma and marginalisation than a homeless person with psychosis and amphetamine use. A person still operating in a high status role may have greater capacity to conceal his/her mental health–substance use problems and their impact. Although financial and social resources may offer some protection from stigma, some aspects and types of mental health–substance use problems will attract stigma regardless of the person's situation.

Government activities sometimes attempt to tackle stigma towards selected groups. For example, campaigns to demystify mental disorders seek to provide the public with education, and to normalise disorders by highlighting their frequency, and having well-known personalities reveal and discuss their mental health condition publicly. Other actions may aim to inflate stigma. For example, 'tough on drugs' stances, anti-smoking campaigns and policies, and 'just say no' campaigns, bank on the deterrent value of stigma in an attempt to control behaviour and reduce demand for substances. However, the flipside of these approaches is the increase in the stigma levelled at those individuals who have not been successfully deterred. In the case of nicotine use, many in the older generation started smoking before health risks were well known and, heavily dependent, may now be experiencing serious health consequences. Such people are unlikely to change their behaviour even in the face of graphic advertising, which in turn strengthens community stigma against smoking.

The person, their family and stigma

Stigma may be directed at the self, impacting on the person's view of and beliefs about themselves. They may see themselves as unworthy of help, respect and social inclusion, and as a result isolate themselves further and exacerbate the existing mental health–substance use problems.

People may seek to reduce their own self-directed stigma by judging another mental health and/or substance use problem group or group of behaviours, with beliefs such as *'I'm not as bad as . . .'*, or *'I don't have a problem as I don't . . .'*. A person with depression and alcohol dependence may *'hate druggies'* and *'never touch the stuff'* (i.e. illicit drugs), and seek reassurance that they are not 'crazy'. They may identify that they never lose control when they drink, and focus on the differences between their own behaviour and that of a stereotypic 'alcoholic'. Similarly, injecting drug users may focus on the behaviours they use to keep themselves safe from the potential risks of this method of substance use. Costain interviewed people with schizophrenia who regularly used cannabis and found that the majority did not identify that they had a mental disorder and many believed their use of cannabis had a positive impact on them.[5] While thought disorder may play a role in their perception, these beliefs would offer some protection against stigma to the self.

Family and friends are not immune to the experience of, or the use of, stigma. They may marginalise the person within their own family or friendship network by focusing on their differences, their problems and the difficulties they cause for the family. Perceived stigma towards the family from others may result in family members 'forcing the issue', and result in pushing the person out of the family or into treatment.

Family may perceive judgement from their own peer group, or receive 'helpful advice' on how they 'should' handle the situation with their relative. If greatly involved in the person's care, they may have to deal with health and legal systems, as well as expressed or unexpressed judgements that they are partly responsible for causing or maintaining the situation. Should they choose to remove themselves from a close or carer relationship, they may then face stigma regarding their 'abandonment' of the person.

Impact of and response to stigma

The process of stigma and marginalisation can bring about social isolation should the person be rejected from employment, friendship groups, activities and even family. One study suggests that the impact of stigma may persist after successful treatment, particularly with regard to contribution to the person's remaining symptoms of depression.[6] This contribution to their mood may be as strong as the impact of stress and social factors, such as social support, mastery, stressful life events or chronic stressors. In studies examining integrated treatment for mental health–substance use problems, while there is a significant decline in depressive symptoms, depression often does not return to a non-clinical level.[7,8] This may be related to losses they have experienced (family, friends, jobs, roles) and/or the impact of stigma in regaining esteem and functioning in their own and others' eyes.

Room describes the process of marginalisation as it can occur in people with substance use problems.[9] The pattern of substance use becomes the 'primary deviance'. This results in negative social evaluation, which can start the process of marginalisation or exclusion by others. The affected person may then link in with other marginalised users, forming a 'mutually supportive counterculture', which can result in further marginalisation for the members through 'secondary deviance'. For example, consider the person with alcohol dependence who lives alone and is generally alone except for the time they spend at the pub with other heavy drinkers. People with severe psychosis may only interact with other people with similar problems, and this may be encouraged by services that provide the person with a social network of similar people (for example, group housing and psychiatric rehabilitation services).

People may cope with stigma through changing their behaviour, with the aim of protecting themselves from further rejection. This may be by secrecy (not revealing their past or present mental health–substance use problem) or withdrawal, which can then lead to further isolation.[6] Others may choose the 'less bad' option – for example, attributing their behaviour to their substance use so as not to be labelled as 'crazy'.

Day-to-day life: the family
Mental health–substance use problems can individually affect the family, the individual's perception of their family, and their role and acceptance within that group. Once mental health–substance use problems exist, relatives may place more responsibility on the individual for their mental health problems. It is suggested that relatives perceive the individual with mental health–substance use problems to have more control over the causes of their psychiatric symptoms than do the relatives of people with severe mental disorder alone – the more severe the symptoms, the greater the perceived responsibility.[10] On the other hand, individuals with mental health–substance use problems have expressed lower family satisfaction and greater desire for family treatment than those with severe mental disorder alone.[11]

The impact of the mental health–substance use problems on the family will vary depending on:
➤ the position within the family (child, parent, sibling)
➤ the perceived past and present role (the 'sick relative', the 'breadwinner', the 'housewife/husband', the 'good' or the 'problem' child)
➤ how long the condition has been present (for example, schizophrenia emerging in adolescence with coexisting cannabis use versus depression and alcohol dependence emerging in midlife)
➤ the physical and psychological impact of the conditions
➤ the past and present family dynamics
➤ the behaviours of themselves and their family members.

Any illness is stressful for a family and can significantly affect the family dynamic. Existing tensions may be exacerbated and new ones arise. Old patterns of behaviour may be disrupted and over time new ones will emerge which may serve to either bring the family closer or further apart as a unit.

In some situations, life may become risky for family members. While severe mental disorder alone does not result in a higher risk of violent behaviour, it can if combined with medication non-compliance and substance use.[12] Women living with men with alcohol use problems have been found to be more likely to experience victimisation, injury, mood disorders, anxiety disorders and poorer health. They can experience more life stressors, lower mental/psychological quality of life and greater rates of alcohol use disorders.[13] On the other hand, people with severe mental disorder are up to 11 times more likely to be victims of violent crime,[14] with the risk increasing with coexisting substance use,[15] rendering them an extremely vulnerable group. For family, the experience of seeing their loved one become a victim of violence can be extremely distressing.

With regard to children, while mental health–substance use problems do not necessarily mean that someone will be a poor parent, children whose parents have mental health–substance use problems may be at greater risk of short- and longer-term difficulties. This is the case when compared to children of parents without mental health–substance use problems, and also those whose parents have one of the problems in isolation. Children exposed to paternal mental health problems, substance use and domestic violence were at greater risk of behaviour problems when young,[16] and depression, alcohol and drug problems, and smoking in adulthood,[17] with the risk increasing with the greater number of the three issues faced by the parents.

Families of people with mental health–substance use problems are often their primary and only support. Support may be given financially, emotionally, or with activities of daily living. Financial support may prevent the person from suffering the negative consequences of poverty. It has been suggested that family and informal caregiver support was related to a greater reduction in substance use during treatment in people with schizophrenia, and that financial support had a greater impact on reducing their use than did the amount of informal care given.[18]

Carers of people with any illness are at increased risk of stress, burn-out and their own mental health problems, particularly depression symptoms. However, a positive relationship with the individual can be a protective factor.[19]

Work and money

Excessive use of any substance can result in a high financial cost. For people with severe mental disorder who smoke, as much as one third of income may be spent on cigarettes.[20] Cost includes the financial outlay of purchase, often at the expense of other commodities, as well as reduced earning potential. Disadvantaged groups, including those with severe mental health–substance use problems, will have compromised earning ability, potentially having greater difficulty gaining and keeping employment. People who start using cannabis during adolescence are likely to have lower income, and lower levels of employment and degree attainment at age 25, even when coexisting mental health problems are taken into account.[21]

Furthermore, any health problem requiring medical intervention brings with it additional costs. This may just be medication and other interventions for the mental health problem. However, mental health–substance use problems result in greater risk of many physical health problems, which bring additional financial burden.

Poverty has a greater impact on the individual and society than simply compromising day-to-day life. Poverty may be the factor that links mental disorder with social problems, such as crime, unemployment and homelessness.[22] The existence of poverty may be associated with lack of education, problems with employment, substance use and lack of positive social attachments. For people with schizophrenia in treatment, financial assistance from the family served to help them have greater reductions in their substance use compared to those without this assistance,[18] challenging the idea that any extra money would likely be spent on drugs. Financial assistance had a greater impact than did other forms of assistance. It was suggested that people with severe mental disorder can better address their substance use problems once basic economic needs are met.

Although family members or partners may provide financial support, and some people are able to access government benefits, these supports may be inadequate or unavailable. Some people may be forced to resort to criminal activities, such as theft, dealing or prostitution to support their day-to-day expenses, including purchasing the substance. Over half of women and almost one fifth of men entering US substance use treatment programmes reported a history of prostitution.[23] Prostitution has been found to be linked to mental and physical health problems, such as:

➤ HIV and other blood-borne and sexually transmitted infections
➤ physical injuries
➤ gynaecological problems
➤ depression
➤ post-traumatic stress disorder
➤ increased likelihood of suicide attempts.

People with severe mental disorder are more likely to be victims of violent crime,[14] which would be exacerbated by becoming involved in criminal activities and networks.

Even among those for whom poverty is not the norm, mental health–substance use problems can nevertheless significantly affect their financial situation and work life. Reduced discretionary spending can impact on quality of life and leisure activities. This may then adversely affect their mental health symptoms and potential for change. For example, a person with depression and alcohol use may be unable to afford to enrol in a course, go on a holiday, update their car or engage in many other pleasurable activities. Due to these limitations it may be more challenging for them to reverse the spiral of inactivity that can occur with depression or replace the recreational component of alcohol. Productivity at work may be affected; sick leave may rise, reducing likelihood of promotion or advancement. This may in turn diminish the person's self-worth, perpetuating the problem.

Medical illness and the medical system

Long-term substance use places a person at increased risk of physical health problems. In addition, mental disorders and the treatments for them can also adversely affect health. This places people with mental health–substance use problems at increased risk of long-term health problems. Acute health risks include:

➤ overdose
➤ injury while intoxicated
➤ self-harm
➤ suicide attempt
➤ medication side-effects.

Substance use places people with severe mental disorder at higher risk of diseases, such as HIV and hepatitis,[24] while people with chronic pain with a history of mental health or substance use problems are twice as likely to be on opioid therapy.[25] Substance use may affect the efficacy of medications provided or the symptoms experienced may be worsened by the mental health problem (e.g. increased perception of pain in a person with depression).

People with mental health–substance use problems may be treated differently within the medical system. Their medical problems may be misdiagnosed as psychiatric or drug and alcohol issues; treatment may be refused (e.g. not being eligible for a transplant unless abstinent) or adjusted; and stigma from medical staff, other individuals, or the individual themselves may be encountered (e.g. the smoker brought the lung cancer on themselves). The individual and/or their family may need to resort to less socially appropriate behaviours to get the person medical attention, with 'the squeaky wheel getting the oil', which may serve to increase existing tension between the individual and the professional.

All of these factors can make an already stressful and challenging situation – being medically unwell – more difficult. The person may feel unworthy of treatment; they or their family may experience anger at the system; or their medical situation may be more confusing and difficult for the professions to determine because of the impact of the mental health–substance use problems, adding to the person's uncertainty. Labelling of the individual may be less informed but pervasive; for example, a psychiatric diagnosis written by a professional in the medical file may then continue to be referred to throughout that person's current and future admissions or appointments regardless of whether there is sufficient evidence to support the diagnosis. This may serve to reinforce and increase the stigma against the individual.

Quality of life and other considerations
The issues outlined above, stigma, the family and financial considerations, all impact on a person's perception of themselves, their role and their quality of life. Mental health–substance use problems seem to have a greater impact on outcome and quality of life than substance use alone. A comparison of different mental health–substance use groups revealed that quality of life was lowest in people with both alcohol dependence and depression and highest in those with alcohol dependence alone.[26] Female methamphetamine users with depression have been found to have lower self-esteem and higher use than those without depression.[27] Similarly, in young people with mental health problems, those with coexisting substance use problems had poorer psychosocial functioning, and continued problems with symptoms and functioning at six months.[28]

PART 2: THE JOURNEY TO CHANGE
There may come a point where a person chooses to change their substance use, or seek treatment for their mental health problem. However, many people, in some cases the majority, do not seek or receive treatment for a variety of reasons, systemic and personal. Just as living with mental health–substance use problems involves not only the individual but their family and wider society, these factors also impact on the change journey.

Barriers to treatment
Systemic barriers
Most people with mental health–substance use problems do not receive any treatment,[29] and at least in the United States, people with mental health–substance use problems are more likely to receive mental health treatment even if they have substance use problems alone.[30] Even if treatment is sought, it is not necessarily going to be available or adequate for a range of reasons, including:

➤ cost
➤ failure to perceive need for services
➤ shortage of trained providers
➤ faulty diagnoses
➤ lack of clinical consensus regarding best treatment.[31,32]

Barriers to treatment vary from country to country.[33] Low expectations of people with mental health–substance use problems can be a significant barrier to change. While smoking has been banned in public hospitals in Australia for some years, for instance, up until recently, there was no such ban in psychiatric units. Smoking has often been seen as 'the least of their worries' and smoking bans as unnecessary hardships for people in psychiatric institutions. Such attitudes are likely to have been associated with the continuing high rates of smoking among people with mental health problems.

Within treatment services there may be confusion or lack of confidence in dealing with coexisting conditions, or different combinations of conditions. People with mental health–substance use problems may be seen as difficult to treat, and certainly it appears that there is less treatment success than in people with one condition alone.[3] The individual themselves may also feel the available system is inappropriate or inadequate. For example, amphetamine users may not see themselves as 'fitting in' with people with alcohol dependences, and staff may be less confident in dealing with the individual as they may be more 'edgy' and have more mental health symptoms than alcohol users.

The metaphor of the 'comorbidity roundabout' to describe the challenges these individuals face has been suggested.[34] The individual with mental health–substance use problems is seen as the driver and the system as the roundabout. Mental health–substance use may lead the driver to become stuck on the roundabout as they:

> consider a range of internal and external conditions (knowledge about services, support from family, friends, health providers, motivation to change, etc.), account for their vehicle's characteristics (other conditions and demands, including social/legal/financial issues), keep their travel itinerary in mind (plans for change including treatment) and navigate through the many detours and dead-ends that they may confront (eligibility for services, accessibility of treatments, etc.).[34]

For the individual, dealing with these factors can be overwhelming, confusing and even demoralising. Negative experiences may result in refusal to consider future assistance and lead the person to feel more vulnerable and untreatable.

Personal barriers

On a personal level, Room commented that '*entering treatment for alcohol or drug prob-lems is potentially humiliating evidence of failure in self-management*'.[9] The person may have believed that the problem would get better on its own, to recover from depression they just needed to 'chin up' and get over it, and alcohol was just a method of coping with the stress in their lives at the moment – they could stop at any time. Seeking treat-ment may be akin to admitting failure or weakness. Coping strategies to protect the person against personal and social stigma, such as secrecy, denial and withdrawal, are essentially undermined by the process of seeking treatment. Being assessed and labelled by a professional, while being beneficial for the purpose of treatment, will often lead to negative stigma effects.[6] A label once given never really goes away, and the person can never return to the point at which their mental health–substance use problems were undefined and, therefore, potentially non-existent.

Motivational forces drive behaviour. While it may appear that there are only negative consequences of a behaviour, or that negatives should outweigh the positives of engaging in the behaviour, the person engaging in the behaviour may see things very differently. The perceived positive effect of alcohol in reducing the distress resulting from post-traumatic stress disorder symptoms in a war veteran may continue to be more important than his wife's distress at his behaviour when intoxicated. While the distress continues to be relieved by the alcohol, treatment for the post-traumatic stress disorder may not be seen to be important. The euphoria of a manic episode compared to the experience of being on antipsychotic medication, and a belief that cannabis helps keep hallucinations under control,[5] may encourage cannabis use and discourage medication compliance. Psychological symptoms of withdrawal (anxiety, depression, irritability) may be inter-preted by the person as a symptom of their mental health problem and used as evidence that the substance helps control their mental health problem. This may serve to increase the perceived positives of the substance use.

Along similar lines, the perceived losses resulting from changing the mental health–substance use may be seen as too great. The substance may have taken on a life and role of its own for the person – always there when needed, never judging. The temporary relief of suffering or pain from loneliness, boredom, insomnia, physical trauma, medi-cal and psychiatric disorders may be too difficult to give up, and if the person has not had the chance to develop alternate coping strategies they may see no viable option for dealing with these experiences. Treatment for anxiety disorders is inherently anxiety provoking, confronting and challenging the person who usually seeks to avoid the anxi-ety experience through substance use.

It may be that the person does not recognise the problem. This may be described as denial, or the 'precontemplation' phase (the initial 'stage of change' where the person believes that the identified behaviour, be it substance use, physical inactivity, medica-tion non-compliance, unhealthy eating and so on, is not a problem and does not require treatment[35] – *see* Book 4, Chapter 6). Alternatively, it may be that the person does not have the capacity to recognise the problem, for example, in a person with psychosis, or alcohol or benzodiazepine use by a person with dementia. The direct impact of the men-tal health–substance use problems may also affect personal resources. Cognitive deficits experienced by people with psychotic disorders may affect their judgement and problem solving, and excessive substance use may also affect people's cognition. Depression can impact on motivation, while fear and anxiety may result in avoidance.

A change in behaviour will impact not only on the person, but on their network. For example, a change in the substance use of a smoker or alcohol user whose partner and network also smoke or drink would bring a number of challenges to all involved. A change to the individual's behaviour may also affect their position and role in their social group. A cannabis user may support their use by dealing in the substance. Their primary social network may consist of other users that they may supply, or their suppliers. Thus, the person may have found a role within the network that marginalisation and poverty has guided them to, and that role may be inextricably linked with their substance use. They may be seen as too risky to employ in 'normal' society, however appreciated and valued within their network. For some people the potential loss of this role and network may far outweigh any benefits of changing their use.

In general, it is important to remember that any change, even a positive one, can involve overcoming significant barriers and a willingness to risk the experience of loss. Recognising these losses associated with change and understanding the positives of the 'problem' behaviour can assist in supporting the person through their change.

CONCLUSIONS

Living with mental health–substance use problems has a greater impact on the individual, their family, society and professionals than having one of the conditions in isolation.

KEY POINT 8.1

Mental health–substance use problems can be seen on a continuum. The challenges of living with both can span across family life, financial and work roles and physical health.

Mental health–substance use conditions are highly stigmatised. Marginalisation resulting from stigma may result in social isolation and poverty, processes that may increase the negative impact of the conditions on the person. It may act as a barrier to access to, and acceptance of, adequate treatment for the conditions.

The majority of people with mental health–substance use problems do not receive any treatment due to a range of perceived and actual barriers to care. Understanding these barriers, including the potential losses of changing their behaviour, can lead to a greater ability to assist that person through these changes.

REFLECTIVE PRACTICE EXERCISE 8.1

Time: 20 minutes
Take time to reflect on the following. Write down your thoughts, your feelings, your beliefs.
- Is psychoactive substance use on a continuum? If so, can you explain why?
- What substances are used by people?
- What is stigma?
- How might stigma affect a person with mental health–substance use problems in

their day-to-day life? (Consider family, social network, work/school, medical and mental health services.)
* What is meant by primary and secondary deviance?
* What personal barriers to change may a person with mental health–substance use problems face?

REFERENCES

1 Kessler RC, Chiu WT, Demler O, *et al.* Prevalence, severity, and comorbidity of 12-month DSM-IV disorders in the National Comorbidity Survey Replication. 2005; *Arch Gen Psychiatry.* **62**: 617–27.

2 Havassay BE, Alvidrez J, Owen KK. Comparisons of patients with comorbid psychiatric and substance use disorders: implications for treatment and service delivery. *Am J Psychiatry.* 2004; **161**: 139–45.

3 Johnson J. Cost-effectiveness of mental health services for persons with a dual diagnosis: a literature review and the CCMHCP. The cost-effectiveness of community mental health care for single and dually diagnosed project. *J Subst Abuse Treat.* 2000; **18**: 119–27.

4 Room R, Rehm J, Trotter RT II, *et al.* Cross-cultural views on stigma, valuation, parity and societal values towards disability. In Üstün TB, Chatterji S, Bickenback, JE, *et al.*, editors. *Disability and Culture: universalism and diversity.* Seattle, WA: Hogrefe & Huber; 2001.

5 Costain WF. The effects of cannabis abuse on the symptoms of schizophrenia: patient perspectives. *Int J Ment Health Nurs.* 2008; **17**: 227–35.

6 Link BG, Struening EL, Rahav M, *et al.* On stigma and its consequences: Evidence from a longitudinal study on men with dual diagnoses of mental illness and substance abuse. *J Health Soc Behav.* 1997; **38**: 177–90.

7 Kay-Lambkin FJ, Baker AL, Lewin TJ, *et al.* Computer-based psychological treatment for comorbid depression and problematic alcohol and/or cannabis use: a randomized controlled trial of clinical efficacy. *Addiction.* 2009; **104**: 378–88.

8 Baker AL, Bucci S, Lewin TJ, *et al.* Cognitive-behavioural therapy for substance use disorders in people with psychotic disorders. *B J Psychiatry.* 2006; **188**: 439–48.

9 Room R. Stigma, social inequality and alcohol and drug use. *Drug Alcohol Rev.* 2005; **24**: 143–55. p. 152.

10 Niv N, Lopez SR, Glynn SM, *et al.* The role of substance use in families' attributions and affective reactions to their relative with severe mental illness. *J Nerv Ment Dis.* 2007; **195**: 307–14.

11 Dixon L, McNary S, Lehman A. Substance abuse and family relationships of persons with severe mental illness. *Am J Psychiatry.* 1995; **152**: 456–8.

12 Swartz MS, Swanson JW, Hiday VA, *et al.* Violence and severe mental illness: the effects of substance abuse and non-adherence to medication. *Am J Psychiatry.* 1998; **155**: 226–31.

13 Dawson DA, Grant BF, Chou BF, *et al.* The impact of partner alcohol use problems on women's physical and mental health. *J Stud Alcohol Drugs.* 2007; **68**: 66–75.

14 Teplin LA, McClelland GM, Abram KM, *et al.* Crime victimization in adults with severe mental illness: comparison with the National Crime Victimization Survey. *Arch Gen Psychiatry.* 2005; **62**: 911–21.

15 Hiday VA, Swartz MS, Swanson JW, *et al.* Criminal victimization of persons with severe mental illness. *Psychiatr Serv.* 1999; **50**: 62–8.

16 Whitaker RC, Orzol SM, Kahn RS. Maternal mental health, substance use, and domestic violence in the year after delivery and subsequent behaviour problems in children at age 3 years. *Arch Gen Psychiatry.* 2006; **63**: 551–60.

17 Felitti VJ, Anda RF, Nordenberg D, *et al.* Relationship of childhood abuse and household

dysfunction to many of the leading causes of death in adults: the Adverse Childhood Experiences (ACE) Study. *Am J Prev Med.* 1998; **14**: 245–58.

18 Clark RE. Family support and substance use outcomes for persons with mental illness and substance use disorders. *Schizophr Bull.* 2001; **27**: 93–101.

19 Pickett SA, Cook JA, Cohler BJ, *et al.* Positive parent/adult child relationships: impact of severe mental illness and caregiver burden. *Am J Orthopsychiatry.* 1997; **67**: 220–30.

20 Lasser K, Boyd JW, Woolhandler S, *et al.* Smoking and mental illness: a population-based prevalence study. *JAMA.* 2000; **284**: 2606–10.

21 Fergusson DM, Boden JM. Cannabis use and later life outcomes. *Addiction.* 2008; **103**: 969–76.

22 Draine J, Salzer MS, Culhane DP, *et al.* Role of social disadvantage in crime, joblessness, and homelessness among persons with serious mental illness. *Psychiatr Serv.* 2002; **53**: 565–73.

23 Burnette ML, Lucas E, Ilgen M, *et al.* Prevalence and health correlates of prostitution among patients entering treatment for substance use disorders. *Arch Gen Psychiatry.* 2008; **65**: 337–44.

24 Devieux JG, Malow R, Lerner BG, *et al.* Triple jeopardy for HIV: substance using severely mentally ill adults. *J Prev Interv Community.* 2007; **33**: 5–18.

25 Sullivan MD, Edlund MJ, Zhang L, *et al.* Association between mental health disorders, problem drug use, and regular prescription opioid use. *Arch Intern Med.* 2006; **166**: 2087–93.

26 Saatcioglu O, Yapici A, Cakmak D. Quality of life, depression and anxiety in alcohol dependence. *Drug Alcohol Rev.* 2008; **27**: 83–90.

27 Semple SJ, Zians J, Strathdee SA, *et al.* Psychosocial and behavioural correlates of depressed mood among female methamphetamine users. *J Psychoactive Drugs.* 2007; **Suppl 4**: 353–66.

28 Baker KD, Lubman DI, Cosgrave EM, *et al.* Impact of co-occurring substance use on 6 month outcomes for young people seeking mental health treatment. *Aust N Z J Psychiatry.* 2007; **41**: 896–902.

29 Wang PS, Aguilar-Gaxiola S, Alonso J, *et al.* Use of mental health services for anxiety, mood and substance disorders in 17 countries in the WHO world mental health surveys. *Lancet.* 2007; **370**: 841–50.

30 Harris, KM, Edlund MJ. Use of mental health care and substance abuse treatment among adults with co-occurring disorders. *Psychiatr Serv.* 2005; **56**: 954–9.

31 Drake RE, Wallach MA. Dual diagnosis: 15 years of progress. *Psychiatr Serv.* 2000; **51**: 1126–9.

32 Ridgely MS, Goldman HH, Willenbring M. Barriers to the care of persons with dual diagnoses: organizational and financing issues. *Schizophr Bull.* 1990; **16**: 123–32.

33 Sareen J, Jagdeo A, Cox BJ, *et al.* Perceived barriers to mental health service utilisation in the United States, Ontario, and the Netherlands. *Psychiatr Serv.* 2007; **58**: 357–64.

34 Kay-Lambkin FJ, Baker AL, Lewin TJ. The 'co-morbidity roundabout': a framework to guide assessment and intervention strategies and engineer change among people with co-morbid problems. *Drug Alcohol Rev.* 2004; **23**: 407–23.

35 Prochaska JO, DiClemente CC. Stages and processes of self-change of smoking: toward an integrative model of change. *J Consult Clin Psychol.* 1983; **51**: 390–5.

TO LEARN MORE

Baker A, Velleman R, editors. *Clinical Handbook of Co-existing Mental Health and Drug and Alcohol Problems.* London: Routledge; 2007.

Mills KL, Deady M, Proudfoot H, *et al. Guidelines on the Management of Co-occurring Alcohol and Other Drug and Mental Health Conditions in Alcohol and Other Drug Treatment Settings.* NDARC; 2009. Available at: http://ndarc.med.unsw.edu.au/NDARCWeb.nsf/page/Comorbidity+Guidelines (accessed 11 March 2010).

CHAPTER 9

Working with people with mental health–substance use

Kim T Mueser

INTRODUCTION

Working with people with mental health–substance use problems is common in the helping profession. The complexity of the challenges facing people with mental health–substance use problems can be daunting for the individual and professional alike. Only by understanding the nature and scope of the problem(s) can professionals be fully prepared to work with, and treat, the multiple problems experienced by people with mental health–substance use problems. In this chapter, we begin with a brief review of the importance of working with mental health–substance use issues in people who present with both problems, including the scope of the problem. The chapter focuses on strategies for working effectively with people who have mental health–substance use problems. We conclude by focusing on how the professional can be optimistic, hopeful, energised and effective in their efforts to help the individual with these challenging problems, develop worthwhile, meaningful and rewarding lives.

THE IMPORTANCE OF TREATING MENTAL HEALTH–SUBSTANCE USE PROBLEMS

People with mental health problems who use substances experience a wide range of negative consequences of their substance use.[1] Some of the most common ones include:
➤ relapses and re-hospitalisations
➤ depression, demoralisation, suicide
➤ housing instability and homelessness
➤ legal problems
➤ health problems
➤ family conflict and other social problems
➤ difficulties managing money
➤ non-adherence to medication and other treatments.

Similarly, individuals with substance use problems experience a multitude of negative outcomes when their use is complicated by mental health problems. For example, mental health problems in people who use substances are associated with:

➤ more severe substance use
➤ greater impaired psychosocial functioning
➤ poorer engagement and higher rate of drop out from treatment
➤ more rapid relapses
➤ greater difficulty participating in and benefiting from addiction self-help groups.

Substance use problems in mental health populations are common, as are mental health problems in people receiving substance use treatment.[2,3] In general, the more severe the psychiatric illness, the higher the rate of substance use problems, and the more severe the substance use, the more likely the person is to have a mental health problem. Some basic facts about mental health–substance use problems are summarised in Box 9.1.

BOX 9.1 Basic facts about mental health–substance use problems

- Mental health–substance use problems are the norm rather than the exception.
- Lack of recognition and treatment of mental health–substance use problems is associated with worse outcomes.
- Denial and minimisation of mental health–substance use problems are common.
- Mental health–substance use problems are often missed and not treated because these problems are not fully explored with the individual.
- Not all substance use in people with mental health problems is due to self-medication of symptoms; other explanations include:
  - facilitating socialisation
  - having fun
  - fighting boredom
  - escaping problems
  - having something to look forward to.
- People with mental health problems are more sensitive to the effects of modest amounts of substances, due to the psychobiological vulnerability that underlies their psychiatric disorder.
- Individuals with mental health problems who are most likely to have substance use issues include people who are:
  - men
  - younger
  - single
  - less educated
  - related to family members with a history of substance use.

Considering the wide range of problems each creates when treating the other, it is crucial that professionals are aware of the nature of mental health–substance use problems in the individual they treat.

WORKING EFFECTIVELY WITHIN MENTAL HEALTH–SUBSTANCE USE

The most important ingredient to effective care for people with mental health–substance use problems is the integration of the treatment of both into a seamless package.[4] The focus of work needs to be on helping the individual overcome his/her problems and achieving personal goals, rather than narrowly treating one or the other. *Integrated treatment* of mental health–substance use problems is most successful when one professional, or team of professionals working together, assumes full responsibility for treating mental health–substance use together, and for integrating the treatments. In addition, there are several factors that are critical to successful treatment of persons with mental health–substance use problems. We review these factors below.

The therapeutic relationship

Changes in mental health–substance use problems occur in the context of a therapeutic relationship between the individual and professional (*see* also Book 4, Chapter 2). Therefore, the professional's first priority is to establish a *therapeutic relationship* or *working alliance* with the individual, and to demonstrate caring and concern. Work on fostering the individual's insight into his/her problems, and motivation to work on them, can proceed after a good relationship has been established.

The therapeutic relationship can be defined by and includes three different components.

1 Agreement between the individual and the professional on the goals of treatment.
2 Agreement on the tasks used to achieve those goals.
3 The bond between the two individuals.[5] Establishing person-centred goals is a good method for beginning a working relationship. This involves understanding the:
   — nature of the individual's life
   — ways in which he/she is satisfied with that life
   — ways in which the individual would like his/her life to change.

The following types of questions are examples of how to begin a dialogue aimed at eliciting person-centred goals to work on together.

➤ **What's important in your life?** Probe for areas, such as close relationships, meaningful work, parenting, religion/spirituality, quality of living environment, artistic expression.
➤ **What things are you satisfied with in your life?**
➤ **What things would you like to change in your life?**
➤ **What are the barriers of change for you?**
➤ **If all of your problems were to suddenly go away, how would your life be different?**
➤ **What would you be doing now that you're not currently doing?**

Establishing a strong working relationship with the person is important to achieving long-term treatment goals. Motivation to work on problems that interfere with goals often waxes and wanes over time. If a strong working relationship is maintained, this relationship can help sustain working together even during fluctuations in the individual's motivation to work on mental health–substance use problems.

Ultimately, the most powerful tool the professional has to establish, and maintain, in a working relationship is the ability to instil hope for change. It is through this hope that people are able to marshal the efforts needed to change the long ingrained personal habits and attitudes. Providing a message of hope and optimism, and believing that each person is inherently capable of change, can be powerful for individuals who themselves may have no hope for their own future.[6]

SELF-ASSESSMENT EXERCISE 9.1

Time: 20 minutes

Consider the comprehensive assessment from the physical, psychological, emotional, social and spiritual aspects.

- What information would you, as the professional, need from this individual to guide you to effective intervention and treatment?

Comprehensive assessment

Comprehensive assessment of problems related to mental health–substance use is of fundamental importance to guiding effective treatment. The most common reason why mental health–substance use problems are not observed and treated in clinical settings is that professionals simply do not ask the questions necessary to identify the problems. Consequently, undetected problems often interfere with the effective treatment and attainment of goals. A comprehensive assessment is important not only to identifying all the pertinent problems that the individual is experiencing, but to better understanding the person's life, potential areas of change, personal strengths, and other important resources, such as social support (*see* Book 5, Chapter 9).

Taking a comprehensive assessment leads naturally to treatment planning, which is primarily informed by the specific goals of treatment agreed upon early in the therapeutic relationship. People may or may not present for treatment of their mental health or substance abuse problems; in either case, functional goals need to be identified that are the focus of collaboration between the person and professional, with attention to mental health–substance use problems as barriers to achieving goals. The identification of functional goals (e.g. improved relationships, ability to return to work) during the assessment can serve as a basis for enhancing motivation to address mental health–substance use problems that interfere with obtaining valued goals.

Comprehensive assessment, intervention and treatment planning are interwoven. Following an initial assessment and identification of goals, a treatment plan is formulated and methods for achieving the goals are identified and implemented. Treatment plans are an ongoing process and, therefore, are constantly reviewed, with troubleshooting conducted to address lack of progress in certain areas, and to establish new goals or next steps towards larger goals when progress is evident. Key points for conducting a comprehensive assessment are summarised in Key Points 9.1.

KEY POINTS 9.1 CONDUCTING A COMPREHENSIVE ASSESSMENT

- Routinely explore mental health–substance use problems in all individuals.
- When enquiring about substance use, begin by asking about past substance use,

and then explore current substance use; people are often more willing to talk about past substance use than current use.

- Be matter of fact when exploring about mental health–substance use problems. Let the individual know that problems in these areas are common and that their exploration is a routine part of intervention and treatment.
- Use standardised self-report measures to screen for the presence of substance use[7-9] or mental health problems.[10,11]
- Don't get bogged down trying to distinguish whether the mental health or substance use problem is 'primary' or 'secondary'; assume that both are 'primary' and require intervention and treatment until you know more.
- Get detailed information about the individual's substance use, including:
  - specific substances used
  - methods of use
  - situations in which substances are used (e.g. social situations, coping with symptoms, etc.)
  - pattern of use (e.g. daily use, bingeing)
  - expectations and perceived motives for use (e.g. feeling relaxed, easier to hang out with others, reduced distress from symptoms).
- Get information about the person's functioning, including the areas of:
  - health (e.g. infectious diseases such as hepatitis C)
  - legal problems (e.g. arrests, pending charges)
  - housing (e.g., stability of housing, independence, quality and safety)
  - family relationships (e.g. amount of contact, support, conflict, satisfaction)
  - other social relationships (e.g. social support, close friends, intimate relationships, satisfaction with relationships)
  - work/school (e.g. competitive or other work, involvement in school, interesting work or school)
  - parenting (e.g. contact with children, meeting parental responsibilities, satisfaction with parenting and desire to improve)
  - distress, well-being (e.g. depression, anxiety, anger, optimism, hope, satisfaction, pleasure)
  - spirituality (e.g. involvement in one's faith, connection with others from same religious community)
  - personal strengths (e.g. determination, creativity, sense of humour, flexibility, specific abilities in areas such as art, music, math, social skills, or interpersonal sensitivity).
- Develop an understanding of the role that substance use plays in the individual's life and potential obstacles to cutting back or stopping substance use.
- Evaluate the individual's motivation to work on substance use problems.
- Take your time; a comprehensive assessment is an ongoing process, and details may change as the professional person's own life picture emerges.

Motivation-based treatment

An old adage in psychotherapy is that the therapist has to start where the individual is, rather than where the professional would like the individual to be (*see* Book 4, Chapter 7;

Book 5, Chapter 11). This means that understanding the individual's current needs and concerns is of paramount importance to establishing a relationship and beginning treatment. Many individuals with mental health and substance use issues who are in treatment are not initially motivated to address these problems. In order to effectively work with the individual, the professional(s) must first focus their attention on addressing the individual's current concerns, with the recognition that motivation to address mental health–substance use problems can be harnessed over the course of treatment as people come to understand their impact on personally valued goals.[13]

Motivation-based treatment requires the professional to be aware of the individual's interest in treatment, and to employ interventions that match his/her motivation, and have the promise of further increasing motivation and commitment to change. It can be useful to conceptualise the process of changing one's behaviour (e.g. use of alcohol or drugs, beginning to exercise regularly, taking medication for mental health problems) as proceeding through a series of stages (*see* Book 4, Chapter 6).[13] During the:

➤ **precontemplation stage** – the individual is not even thinking about changing his/her behaviour
➤ **contemplation stage** – the person is considering changing behaviour, but has not yet committed to change
➤ **preparation stage** – the individual is making plans to change, and determining a specific course of action that he/she hopes will be successful in bringing about the desired change
➤ **action stage** – the person's plan is put into place, and either change takes place as expected or additional plans must be developed and implemented
➤ **maintenance stage** – this stages focuses on retaining the gains made, and avoiding a return or relapse of the undesired behaviours, once the individual has successfully changed his/her behaviour.

These *stages of change* naturally take place in individuals, whether or not they are receiving treatment for specific problems. When people are in treatment, the professional's awareness of the person's stage of change can provide a valuable heuristic to selecting interventions that are appropriate for that particular stage of motivation, and that have potential for helping the person move on to the next stage of change. The concept of the stages of change has been adapted to address the *stages of treatment* that people with a mental health problem go through in the context of receiving treatment that also addresses their substance use problem.[14]

Four different stages of treatment have been identified, including *engagement, persuasion, active treatment,* and *relapse prevention*.[15] The stages of treatment correspond to how the stages of change work in the context of a professional helping relationship, and include treatment options appropriate for the individual's current level of motivation. For example, the first stage of treatment is the engagement stage (*see* Book 5, Chapter 7), because a therapeutic relationship is assumed to be a crucial benefit from treatment. The professional does not assume that the individual is committed to working on specific mental health or substance use issues at this early point in treatment, and therefore, the goal of this stage is to establish a working relationship with the person that instils motivation to meet regularly with the professional to address whatever the individual's pressing concerns are. Examples of possible interventions at this stage include outreach to meet with the person in the community, demonstrating empathy, addressing practical needs (e.g. food, clothing, shelter), and helping to resolve a crisis. Notably absent from the engagement stage of treatment is any attempt to convince the person that he/she has a substance use problem, or to try to change their substance use behaviour. These interventions are more appropriate for the later stages of treatment, namely the persuasion and active treatment stages, respectively.

Awareness of the stages of change, and an understanding of the individual's specific stage of treatment, can optimise the professional's effectiveness in selecting interventions that are appropriate for the person's level of motivation to change. For example, stagewise treatment avoids common problems, such as trying to convince the individual that he/she has a substance use problem (a persuasion stage intervention) before a therapeutic relationship is established (when the person is in the engagement stage), often leading to premature dropout from treatment, or attempting to teach the individual skills for refusing offers to use substances (an active treatment intervention) when no interest has been expressed in changing substance use behaviour (when in the persuasion stage), often leading to poor follow-through on targeted skills. Boxes 9.2, 9.3, 9.4 and 9.5 summarise each of the stages of treatment as applied to substance use problems, including the goal of each stage and examples of interventions that may be used to achieve the goal.

BOX 9.2 Goal, definition, and examples of interventions targeting substance use problems at the engagement stage of treatment

Goal To establish a therapeutic relationship.
Definition Meeting with the individual on a regular basis.
Examples of interventions
- Assertive outreach to meet the individual in the community rather than clinic.
- Providing practical assistance (e.g. food, clothing).
- Resolving a crisis (e.g. housing problem, health problem).
- Providing social network support (e.g. assistance to family).
- Legal constraints (e.g. outpatient commitment to treatment.

BOX 9.3 Goal, definition, and examples of interventions targeting substance use problems at the persuasion stage of treatment

Goal To help the individual recognise substance use as a problem, and commence working on it.
Definition Person begins to reduce substance use, stops using substances, or makes repeated attempts to cut down.
Examples of interventions
- Stabilisation of psychiatric symptoms.
- Individual and family psycho-education about mental health–substance use.
- 'Persuasion groups' designed to provide a safe environment for individuals to explore and share their good and bad experiences using substances, to validate their ambivalence about changing behaviour, and to support each other in changing their substance use habits.

- Rehabilitation to build coping and social skills and alternative leisure activities.
- Motivational interviewing to instil desire to change behaviour by increasing awareness of how it will help the individual achieve personally meaningful goals.

BOX 9.4 Goal, definition, and examples of interventions targeting substance use problems for the active stage of treatment

Goal To reduce substance use and/or attain abstinence.
Definition The person has stopped using substances or has not experienced consistent negative consequences of using for at least six months.
Examples of interventions
- Self-monitoring urges to use or actual use.
- Social skills training to refuse offers to use substances.
- Teaching coping skills to manage cravings or symptoms that precipitate use.
- Self-help groups for substance use.
- Social network support.
- Developing new leisure activities and social relationships to replace those involving substance use.

BOX 9.5 Goals, definitions, and examples of interventions targeting substance use problems at the relapse prevention stage

Goal To prevent relapses and extend recovery to other areas of functioning.
Definition Person avoids relapses of substance use problems and improves functioning in other areas such as social, work, school, parenting, health, or independent living.
Examples of interventions
- Self-help groups for substance use to support sobriety or controlled/normal use.
- Cognitive behavioural and supportive interventions to enhance functioning at work/school, in social relationships, independent living, and health/mental health management.
- Developing a relapse prevention plan to prevent recurrences of substance use problems.

Multiple treatment modalities

There are many different pathways to recovery from mental health–substance use problems. Each person's recovery journey is unique, and the art of being effective is helping the individual find his/her own path. Since there is no single road to recovery, the professional needs to be flexible and aware of the range of different treatment options and modalities that may benefit the individual.

Many people with mental health–substance use problems benefit from group interventions.[16] Such interventions can provide validation and social support for each individual's experience, and help individuals meet some of their social needs in a context not involving the use of substances. Groups can also be a very effective modality for teaching new skills, as individuals get the benefit of learning from, and supporting each other, in the practice of skills.

Some individuals benefit from participating in self-help groups help (*see* Book 4, Chapters 9, 14, 15) – others do not.[17] Self-help groups are an important option to explore with the individual but should never be mandatory as such a requirement is incompatible with the very nature of self. People with schizophrenia in particular often report that self-help groups for substance use may not be helpful because they feel awkward in those groups, they often do not relate to the losses of other group members, and they may occasionally meet with disapproval from other group members because of their use of psychiatric medications.

Although group-based interventions are helpful for many people with mental health–substance use problems, the person often needs to be engaged individually in treatment. Furthermore, some people do not like groups, or are too impaired to participate in them, necessitating individual rather than group treatment. Individual work is also helpful as a supplement to group work. Individual interventions can employ a range of therapeutic methods to address mental health–substance use issues, including motivational interviewing and cognitive behavioural therapy (*see* Book 5, Chapters 11, 12).[18,19]

Many people with mental health–substance use problems either live with, or are in regular contact with, their family members. The relationships between people with mental health–substance use problems and the family are often strained by the substance use problems.[20] Nevertheless, families often provide substantial resources, including time, money and emotional support, in helping their loved one.[21] In addition, the involvement of family members in the lives of people with mental health–substance use problems is associated with a better course of ill health, including a more rapid remission of substance use problems.[22] Therefore, family intervention is an important modality for people with mental health–substance use problems.[23] Family intervention can serve to increase understanding about the nature of mental health–substance use concerns and dilemmas, teaching the principles of treating mental health–substance use problems in order to gain the family's support for the individual's involvement in treatment, facilitate the identification of, and support for, achieving the person's personal recovery goals, and reduce stress and tension in the family through improved understanding, communication and problem-solving skills.[15,24]

In addition to psychotherapeutic treatment modalities, pharmacological treatment should not be neglected (*see* Book 5, Chapter 13). Medications have a critical role to play in the treatment of schizophrenia-spectrum disorders, bipolar disorder and major depression.[25] Without these medications, many individuals would be much less able to benefit from psychosocial treatments. There are also effective medications that target substance use. These medications have been primarily studied in substance use populations, but a growing body of research has demonstrated their beneficial effects in people with mental health–substance use problems.[26] Thus, medications are another critical treatment modality that should be considered in the armamentarium of interventions for addressing mental health–substance use problems.

Some individuals are able to participate in and benefit from community-based services, and experience long-term remission of their substance use problems.[27] Others have difficulty benefiting from similar community-based services, and are highly vulnerable to the temptations and pressures to use substances in their living environments. For these individuals, residential treatment is an important option that can provide the individual with protection from opportunities to use substances in a safe environment in which they can develop better skills for developing their social, living and personal needs. [28] Residential programmes tend to be most effective when they are intermediate or long term in length, and they provide a gradual transition from the residential setting back into the community.

Long-term commitment to improving quality of life

Mental health–substance use problems are often chronic, relapsing conditions. Although long-term remission of one or both occurs, many individuals struggle with these problems throughout much of their lives (*see* Book 6, Chapters 15, 16). Thus, treatment needs to be long term, and guided by the recognition of some mental health–substance use problems are persistent challenges for the individual.

Appreciating the persistent nature of mental health–substance use problems is not tantamount to giving up, or continuing to work with, the person towards recovery. Rather, an understanding of the long-term nature of these problems underscores the importance of not narrowly focusing treatment on mental health–substance use issues, but more broadly seeking to improve the individual's self-determination and the quality and enjoyment of life, despite the continuing challenges they face.[29,30] People with mental health–substance use problems want the same things out of life as we do, for example:

➤ close and rewarding relationships with family members and friends
➤ a safe and comfortable place to live
➤ good health
➤ something meaningful to do with one's time
➤ ways of having fun.

All of these aspects of a good quality of life should be the focus of treatment, with the aim of minimising the effects of mental health–substance use problems on functioning in these areas. Thus, a long-term commitment to treatment is predicated on the fact that mental health–substance use problems are often persistent over time, and that intervention needs to focus broadly on improving quality of life and the management of any persistent mental health or substance use issues.

SELF-CARE FOR THE PROFESSIONAL

Treating individuals with mental health–substance use problems can be a taxing, frustrating experience. For example, it can be painful to develop a helping relationship with someone who continues to engage in self-harming behaviours, such as excessive substance use, or not taking medications that could effectively control psychiatric symptoms. The person may appear unmotivated or unappreciative of the professionals' continued efforts, leading to the perennial question of whether the professional is working harder than the individual.

At the same time, there are tremendous rewards associated with treating people with substance use–mental health problems. With help, and over time, people do recover their lives. However, in order to maintain a helping relationship, professionals must remain optimistic in their work, and convey the sense of the genuine possibility of recovery to every individual with whom they work. We, the professional, need to be sensitive to our own needs in order to make a difference, and to be aware of how our attitudes, and sense of hope, affects the individual with whom they work (*see* Book 2, Chapters 10, 11). Key Points 9.2 summarises some of the helpful strategies we may find helpful in avoiding demoralisation and burn-out, and may help us to remain hopeful and optimistic about the person's ability to overcome his/her concerns and dilemmas.

KEY POINTS 9.2

For professionals to avoid burn-out and demoralisation

- Remember that mental health–substance use problems are genuine. They are no one's fault; mental health–substance use problems run in families and have a biological basis.
- Remind yourself that although co-occurring disorders have a biological basis, they also interact with the person's coping efforts, social supports, and the environment, and thus through collaborative work their outcomes can be improved.
- Note that the individuals who are most difficult to treat often need your help the most.
- Take a collaborative-empirical approach to exploring and implementing different solutions to problems; when one solution doesn't work, try, try again!
- Involve the appropriate intra- and interdisciplinary team(s) in treatment planning and monitoring outcomes. Include the individual, family members and significant other in the person's life; many hands make light work.
- Assume that all individuals have the innate capability to recover.
- Broaden your focus from mental health–substance use issues to helping the person to improve his/her quality of life.
- Remember that most individuals do improve in the long run.
- Always develop a case formulation aimed at understanding what factors maintain the person's mental health–substance use problems and, therefore, need to be addressed in treatment; modify or change your formulation if treatment based on it does not achieve its desired effects.
- Although the individuals' coping efforts may seem ineffective at times, avoid blaming people by remembering that everybody is doing the best they can.

CONCLUSION

Mental health–substance use problems are common. They present significant challenges to all involved – the individual, family and professional. Understanding the lives that people live, and the roles that mental health–substance use problems play in their lives, can lead to effective treatment plans aimed at helping people learn how to develop alternative and more effective ways of getting their needs met. Treatment does work in the long run, but patience and persistence are necessary in the face of slow change and setbacks that are a normal part of the healing process.

All treatment hinges on the relationship between the individual and the professional. Therefore, developing a working alliance is of fundamental importance. Seeking to discover the hopes and dreams that each person harbours within them, and conveying the belief that change is possible, can lead to the identification of treatment goals that serve as the basis for the therapeutic relationship. Maintaining this relationship, and focusing on helping the person achieve personally meaningful goals, is the key to successful collaboration in treatment, and progress along the road to recovery.

REFERENCES

1 Drake RE, Brunette MF. Complications of severe mental illness related to alcohol and other drug use disorders. In: Galanter M, editor. *Recent Developments in Alcoholism: consequences of alcoholism.* New York, NY: Plenum Publishing Company; 1998. pp. 285–99.

2 Kessler RC, Nelson CB, McGonagle KA, *et al.* The epidemiology of co-occurring addictive and mental disorders: implications for prevention and service utilization. *Am J Orthopsychiatry.* 1996; **66**: 17–31.

3 Regier DA, Farmer ME, Rae DS, *et al.* Comorbidity of mental disorders with alcohol and other drug abuse: Results from the Epidemiologic Catchment Area (ECA) study. *JAMA.* 1990; **264**: 2511–18.

4 Minkoff K. An integrated treatment model for dual diagnosis of psychosis and addiction. *Hosp Community Psychiatry.* 1989; **40**: 1031–6.

5 Bordin ES. The generalizability of the psychoanalytic concept of the working alliance. *Psychotherapy Theory, Res Pract.* 1976; **16**: 252–60.

6 Cooper J, Cooper DB. Hope and coping strategies. In: Cooper J, editor. *Stepping into Palliative Care 1: relationships and responses.* 2nd ed. Oxford: Radcliffe Publishing; 2006.

7 Maisto SA, Carey MP, Carey KB, *et al.* Use of the AUDIT and the DAST-10 to identify alcohol and drug use disorders among adults with a severe and persistent mental illness. *Psychol Assess.* 2000; **12**: 186–92.

8 McHugo GJ, Paskus TS, Drake RE. Detection of alcoholism in schizophrenia using the MAST. *Alcohol Clin Exp Res.* 1993; **17**: 187–91.

9 Rosenberg SD, Drake RE, Wolford GL, *et al.* The Dartmouth Assessment of Lifestyle Instrument (DALI): a substance use disorder screen for people with severe mental illness. *Am J Psychiatry.* 1998; **155**: 232–8.

10 Alexander MJ, Haugland G, Lin SP, *et al.* Mental health screening in addiction, corrections and social service settings: validating the MMS. *Int J Addict.* 2008; **6**: 105–19.

11 Carroll JFX, McGinley JJ. A screening form for identifying mental health problems in alcohol/ other drug dependent persons. *Alcohol Treat Q.* 2001; **19**: 33–47.

12 Miller WR, Rollnick S, editors. *Motivational Interviewing: preparing people for change.* 2nd ed. New York, NY: Guilford Press; 2002.

13 Prochaska JO, DiClemente CC. *The Transtheoretical Approach: crossing the traditional boundaries of therapy.* Homewood, IL: Dow-Jones/Irwin; 1984.

14 Osher FC, Kofoed LL. Treatment of patients with psychiatric and psychoactive substance use disorders. *Hosp Community Psychiatry.* 1989; **40**: 1025–30.

15 Mueser KT, Noordsy DL, Drake RE, *et al.* Integrated Treatment for Dual Disorders: a guide to effective practice. New York, NY: Guilford Press; 2003.

16 Mueser KT, Pierce SC. Group treatment for co-existing mental health and drug and alcohol problems. In: Baker A, Velleman R, editors. *Clinical Handbook of Co-existing Mental Health and Drug and Alcohol Problems.* Hove: Routledge; 2007. pp. 96–113.

17 Noordsy DL, Schwab B, Fox L, *et al.* The role of self-help programs in the rehabilitation of persons with severe mental illness and substance use disorders. *Community Ment Health J.* 1996; **32**: 71–81.

18 Barrowclough C, Haddock G, Beardmore R, *et al.* Evaluating integrated MI and CBT for people with psychosis and substance misuse: recruitment, retention and sample characteristics of the MIDAS trial. *Addict Behav.* 2009; **34**: 859–66.

19 Graham HL, Copello A, Birchwood MJ, *et al. Cognitive-behavioural Integrated Treatment (C-BIT): a treatment manual for substance misuse in people with severe mental health problems.* Chichester: John Wiley & Sons; 2004.

20 Salyers MP, Mueser KT. Social functioning, psychopathology, and medication side effects in relation to substance use and abuse in schizophrenia. *Schizophr Res.* 2001; **48**: 109–23.

21 Clark R. Family costs associated with severe mental illness and substance use: a comparison of families with and without dual disorders. *Hosp Community Psychiatry.* 1994; **45**: 808–13.

22 Clark RE. Family support and substance use outcomes for persons with mental illness and substance use disorders. *Schizophr Bull.* 2001; **27**: 93–101.

23 Mueser KT, Glynn SM, Cather C, *et al.* Family intervention for co-occurring substance use and severe psychiatric disorders: participant characteristics and correlates of initial engagement and more extended exposure in a randomized controlled trial. *Addict Behav.* 2009; **34**: 867–77.

24 O'Grady CP, Skinner WJ. *Partnering with Families Affected by Concurrent Disorders.* Toronto, ON: Centre for Addiction and Mental Health; 2007.

25 Schatzberg AF, Cole JO, DeBattista C, editors. *Manual of Clinical Psychopharmacology.* 3rd ed. Washington, DC: American Psychiatric Publishing Group; 2007.

26 Green AI, Noordsy DL, Brunette MF, *et al.* Substance abuse and schizophrenia: pharmacotherapeutic intervention. *J Subst Abuse Treat.* 2008; **34**: 61–71.

27 Xie H, Drake RE, McHugo GJ. The 10-year course of substance use disorder among patients with severe mental illness: an analysis of latent class trajectory groups. *Psychiatr Serv.* 2009; **60**: 804–11.

28 Brunette MF, Mueser KT, Drake RE. A review of research on residential programs for people with severe mental illness and co-occurring substance use disorders. *Drug Alcohol Rev.* 2004; **23**: 471–81.

29 Davidson L, Tondora J, Lawless MS, *et al. A Practical Guide to Recovery-oriented Practice: tools for transforming mental health care.* New York, NY: Oxford University Press; 2009.

30 Ryan RM, Deci EL. Self-determination theory and the facilitation of intrinsic motivation, social development and well-being. *Am Psychol.* 2000; **55**: 68–78.

TO LEARN MORE

Bellack AS, Bennet ME, Gearon JS. *Behavioral Treatment for Substance Abuse in People with Serious and Persistent Mental Illness: a handbook for mental health professionals.* New York: Taylor & Francis; 2007.

Cooper J, Cooper DB. Hope and coping strategies. In: Cooper J, editor. *Stepping into Palliative Care 1: relationship and responses.* Oxford: Radcliffe Publishing; 2006.

Liberman RP. *Recovery from Disability: manual of psychiatric rehabilitation.* Washington, DC: American Psychiatric Press; 2008.

McGovern MP, Drake RE, Merrens MR, *et al. Hazelden Co-occurring Disorders Program: integrated service for substance use and mental health problems.* Center City, MN: Hazelden; 2008.

Mueser KT, Noordsy DL, Drake RE, *et al. Integrated Treatment for Dual Disorders: a guide to effective practice.* New York: Guilford Press; 2003.

Roberts LJ, Shaner A, Eckman TA. *Overcoming Addictions: skills training for people with schizophrenia.* New York: WW Norton; 1999.

Skills, capabilities and professional development: a response framework for mental health–substance use

Carmel Clancy and Adenekan Oyefeso

INTRODUCTION

The increasing occurrence of mental health–substance use is recognised to have reached a critical point in the ability of services to offer an effective and sustained response. Partial explanation of why individual experiencing mental health–substance use problems are challenging services can be explained by the lack of adequate preparation of the professional:

➤ **technically** – evidenced by the absence of specialist knowledge and skills
➤ **organisationally** – demonstrated by lack of collaborative working practices and integrated care systems.

Overarching these deficits is the presence of a negative attitudinal legacy towards individuals who use substances, and how this correlates the professionals' commitment to the treatment and recovery process.[1]

In recent years, greater attention has been given on how best to tackle the challenge in providing services, with the emphasis on treatment effectiveness and best practices. A current view arising from both empirical and anecdotal evidence is to advance a model of integrated treatment.[2] This approach, which has yet to have a consensual operational definition, follows the principle that a person with mental health–substance use problems must be treated as a 'whole person'; their mental health and substance use problems are deemed a single 'entity' bound together. Efforts to treat one problem without addressing the role of the other are considered to be limited and likely to result in poor outcomes.

SELF-ASSESSMENT EXERCISE 10.1

Time: 15 minutes

Think of a person with whom you have engaged who has experienced mental health–substance use problems.

- Was he/she given a diagnosis? If yes, what was it?

- Was he/she treated for two separate conditions?
- Could the intervention/treatment have been improved?
- How could you have improved the situation for that individual?

In response to the principle of integrated treatment, government agencies, health and social care commissioners and treatment service providers in the United Kingdom are beginning to recognise the enormity of the task of providing a care system that is 'fit for purpose'. This places new demands on healthcare systems and consequently the professional charged with caring for these individuals. If the phenomenon that is mental health–substance use is to be addressed effectively, the issue of how best to prepare both current and future professionals in developing their competencies must be a priority.

The expression *'getting the right people with the right skills and competencies in the right place at the right time'* is often used to describe professional planning.[3] While the provision of effective care offered by direct service professionals requires a range of competencies at multiple levels within the service system, the responsibility of ensuring a truly responsive system is not just a matter of developing specific proficiencies. There is a greater need to acknowledge that training, education and related activities, such as support and empowerment, must be part of a wider professional development strategy. Indeed, there are those who suggest that if work related to substance use is to be truly embraced by mental health professionals, such a development can only occur in the presence of a responsive and similarly prepared work environment and shift in organisational culture.[4]

This chapter offers a professional development framework that considers competencies and role development needs required to work with mental health–substance use problems, and individuals, in a system that traditionally has provided two separate care pathways.

GETTING THE RIGHT PEOPLE
Who exactly are the people who are currently providing care to those experiencing mental health–substance use problems? In the UK, current policy on good practice suggests the need to 'mainstream' mental health–substance use care, ultimately making it 'everyone's business'.[5] As part of this strategic response 'mental health–substance use' was stratified into four categories (*see* Figure 10.1) and mapped to treatment services considered the most appropriate to offer care. For example, individuals assessed as experiencing the severe end of the spectrum for both conditions (i.e. High Mental Illness/High Substance Use), or the severe end of mental illness and low end of problematic substance use (i.e. High Mental Illness/Low Substance Use) are best cared for primarily by psychiatric/mental health services (with input from substance use specialists); while those experiencing the severe end of problematic substance use, and low end of mental illness (i.e. High Substance Use/Low Mental Illness), should be treated primarily by specialist substance use services, and finally, individuals considered to be affected by the low end of each condition (Low Mental Illness/Low Substance Use) are better served within primary care services.

In support of this approach, a number of initiatives have been instigated nationally

Low e.g. a dependent drinker who experiences increasing anxiety.	**High** e.g. an individual with schizophrenia who uses cannabis on a daily basis to compensate for social isolation.
Low e.g. a recreational user of 'dance drugs' who has begun to struggle with low mood after weekend use.	**High** e.g. an individual with bipolar disorder whose occasional binge drinking and experimental drug use destabilises their mental health.

FIGURE 10.1 Severity of problematic mental illness and problematic substance use[5]

including the introduction of specialist mental health–substance use professionals, charged with supporting mainstream mental health services; education and training existing teams who are deemed to have greater contact with mental health–substance use problems and individuals (e.g. assertive outreach); and providing basic substance use awareness training to professionals working in community mental health, inpatient, early intervention and crisis resolution services.

While the expectation may be that these professionals are the 'right' people, there is evidence that professionals' working across these settings report varying degrees of preparation. The link between lack of education and training in the area of substance use and counter-productive attitudes has been established.[6–8] In fact, it has been noted that negative attitudes may actively contribute to the development of 'stigmatisation' and subsequent marginalisation. It has been proposed that the majority of professionals, including those working in mental health, hold negative, stereotypical perceptions of illicit drug use, impeding successful therapeutic engagement and management.[9]

Historically, substance use has received low priority in the education of mental health professionals, irrespective of discipline. There are low overall levels of reported training in substance use among professionals, on placement.[10] Of the reported training received, the focus was theoretical rather than clinical. The highest level of reported training was in alcohol use compared to illicit drug and tobacco use. High numbers of respondents reported feeling responsible for helping individuals with substance use difficulties but low numbers actually felt skilled to do so, indicating high levels of awareness without the requisite training.

One report observed that although the majority of psychologists reported working directly with substance using individuals, most had no formal substance use education (74%) or training (54%).[11] Similarly, in a survey of 32 United Kingdom medical schools, training on substance use was patchy and uncoordinated, and was often viewed as a 'specialism'.[12] Average hours dedicated to the subject across the curricula range from 2–14. One study exploring attitudes of the intra- and interdisciplinary teams towards individuals with mental health–substance use problems found differences across disciplines, particularly related to their perceived roles and their perception of the impact of substances on mental health.[13] For example, doctors attributed more importance to the link between substance use and cause of mental illness, compared to other professionals. Social professionals were found to attach less importance to drug and alcohol as a cause of mental illness, and believed it was less important to employ drug screening in the assessment of the individual experiencing psychotic episodes. Psychologists held more therapeutic optimism for these individuals. A specific training needs survey on mental health–substance use training of psychiatrists, psychiatric nurses, substance use nurses and social professionals was undertaken across England.[14] Key findings revealed that 55% of the sample (n = 80), felt inadequately prepared, and when analysed by type of specialism this figure went up to 68% among professionals who described themselves as 'generalists'.

SKILLS AND CAPABILITIES

This brief account of education and training needs attests to the fact that the current level of preparation among professionals is lagging behind projected capacity required to provide effective services. This deficit still persists despite the introduction over the last 10 years of capability frameworks focusing on the knowledge, skills and attitudes needed for mental health professionals to work effectively with individuals affected by substance use. As early as 2001, the Sainsbury Centre for Mental Health 'Capable Practitioner Framework',[15] introduced in response to the National Service Framework for Mental Health,[16] sets out the 'capabilities' needed to implement the recommended treatment for individuals with mental health problems. This was the first document within a UK context to describe specific capabilities related to individuals with mental health–substance use problems:

> The practitioner specialising in work with people with a [mental health–substance use problem] or personality disorder will need to expand their expertise in medical and psychological interventions specific to [these individuals], their knowledge of the social and cultural context of illicit drug taking and the behavioural issues associated with personality disorder. They will need to be capable of:
> ➤ understanding the ethical & legal issues relating to [these individuals]
> ➤ understanding the barriers to care and treatment
> ➤ undertaking the complex assessment and diagnosis of [these individuals]
> ➤ medication management and interactions with illicit drugs and alcohol
> ➤ motivational interviewing
> ➤ applying cognitive and behavioural approaches
> ➤ using strategies to reduce self-harm and other self-destructive behaviour.[15]

Since then, other relevant frameworks have been published, offering specific guidance on the capabilities required for professionals working specifically with individuals who use substances,[17,18] These frameworks represent a consensus on role expectations dependent on the scope of professional practice. For example, one study offers a model that suggests there are three practitioner levels (i.e. core, generalist and specialist), each requiring a different set of capabilities.[18]

1 **Core**, for example Accident and Emergency professionals, police, criminal justice professionals, housing etc., primarily come into contact with mental health–substance using individuals – because they are individuals:
   — 'at risk' of developing long-term mental health / substance use problems
   — with more severe problems who come into contact with 'core professionals' as first point of contact
   — already engaged with other agencies and for whom the 'core professional' is their primary or key professional.

2 **Generalists**, for example mental health social work professionals and nurses, psychologists, psychiatrists, substance use professionals etc., work with mental health–substance use individuals regularly but are not considered to have a 'specific' role with this group. Typically, individuals will have moderate problems associated with their mental health–substance use problems.

3 **Specialists**, for example mental health–substance use professionals, work specifically with individuals with chronic and complex needs related to their mental health–substance use problems. There is also an expectation that this professional takes responsibility to facilitate training in the area of mental health–substance use treatment, and service development.

The term 'capability' is considered to include the following five elements.[15]
1 Performance (i.e. knowledge, skills required).
2 Ethical (i.e. integration of values and social awareness).
3 Reflective (i.e. ability to reflect on practice).
4 Ability to implement evidence-based practice.
5 Commitment to self-development and working with new models of practice.

Adopting this definition, the first section of the Dual Diagnosis Capability Framework[18] outlines five essential values required by professionals in their ability to be effective.
1 **Role legitimacy**: acknowledging that drug and alcohol problems of their individuals are legitimate areas of enquiry and they have a right to intervene.
2 **Therapeutic optimism.**
3 **Acceptance of the uniqueness of the individual.**
4 **A non-judgemental attitude.**
5 **Ability to demonstrate empathy.**

AN ISSUE OF ROLE
Publications, such as the Dual Diagnosis Capability Framework,[18] offer an initial starting point, from which organisations (both treatment providers and their educational partners) can begin to profile the training needs of current employees, and map level 1, 2, 3 job description/roles to the essential mental health–substance use capabilities. As the framework is multi-professional, or indeed, anchored to length of experience, it is yet unclear how these capabilities can be interpreted at the individual practitioner level. Work on therapeutic commitment suggests that working with complex individuals with

drug and alcohol problems demands role support.[19] However, before focusing on role support, there is a need to understand how a 'role' is defined or enacted.

SELF–ASSESSMENT EXERCISE 10.2

Time: 15 minutes
- If can be difficult to define one's job role. Take time to consider, and note down, the defining elements of your current role.
- If you are a 'specialist', what makes your role different from that of the generalist?

The term 'role' has many definitions and is subject to the context in which it is used. For example, role can imply:

> The actions and activities assigned to or required or expected of a person or group,[20] e.g. 'the role of a mental health–substance use professional'; 'the role of an assertive outreach team'.

Role theory is a conceptual framework that defines how individuals behave in social situations and how these behaviours are perceived by external observers. In combining the main theories, the following assumptions in relation to role can be formed:[21]

> ➤ Behaviours are patterned and are characteristic of people within contexts (i.e. behaviours within certain positions dictate specific roles to be performed or require certain patterns of behaviour.
> ➤ Roles are associated with sets of people who share a common identity (e.g. mental health–substance use professionals).
> ➤ People are often aware of roles and to some extent are governed by the fact of their awareness, i.e. expectations.
> ➤ Roles persist in part, because of their consequences (functions) and embedment within larger social systems.
> ➤ People must be taught roles (i.e. socialised), which can be both pleasant and painful.[21]

The above interpretation may in part assist in understanding how underlying values held by professionals who have authority, or the wider cultural values of an organisation, may influence how role development in the area of mental health–substance use is facilitated or hampered. All job roles have two components: formal and informal. The former is associated with explicit role expectations, e.g. job description, while the latter relates to informal expectations or the sub-text of the role, in other words, the unofficial way of doing things. Informal expectations also tend to be implicit and refer to the attitudinal and cognitive features of role performance, and if transgressed can have greater consequences than formal role expectations.[22] Hence role development can be strongly influenced by the professionals' environment and their interactions and observations of co-professionals. As professionals navigate the processes of change there is often a need to explore, refine and often redefine roles.[23] This particularly occurs when individuals are challenged to assume new work patterns or environments (e.g. mental health–substance use). For example, a mental health nurse being asked to undertake a drug and alcohol screening assessment, or employing motivational enhancement techniques that have not been previously considered part of their role.

Role transition
Role transition from generic to specialist has been explored; and noted to be unsettling for experienced professionals changing to specialties, and compounded by moving into emotionally charged areas of practice (e.g. mental health–substance use, hospice care).[22] Unlike newly qualified professionals who report experiencing 'not knowing' due to lack of experience, qualified practitioners who believed they had already acquired a 'set of skills' report feeling 'de-skilled', manifesting as lack of confidence in their abilities on first starting in a new area of practice.[22,24–6] One study suggests that de-skilling can be the outcome of lack of perceived 'specialist' skills; triggered by co-professionals' unrealistic expectations of the newcomer, or lack of acknowledgement of transferable skills.[25] Another study of nurses moving from acute care wards to specialist critical care units reported the importance of knowledge and skill acquisition and its correlation with increased confidence, self-esteem and job performance.[24]

Role development and support
In addition to identifying the 'capabilities' required to work effectively with the mental health–substance use individual, it is important to understand the professional's current stage of role development, especially their transitional point, so that responsive and tailor-designed support can be offered by the organisation. Although three levels of practitioners have been proposed,[18] not all practitioners start from the same position of experience (either technical, emotional or personal).

> **KEY POINT 10.1**
>
> The professional brings to their practice unique aspects of 'self', which influences the work role, and the working interactions as a member of a team, organisation and the community.

When examining role development among nurses who worked in substance use practice, one study identified five stages:[22]
1 Encounter
2 Engagement
3 Stabilisation
4 Competency
5 Mastery.

Each stage of development has its own set of unique characteristics, and expressed the nurses' perception of their capabilities (role adequacy), motivation and emotional expression (how they felt about their performance, or how the environment/individuals made them feel about themselves). The stages, reported as progressive in nature and of variable duration, are influenced by prior experience, access to:

> ➤ specialist substance use training
> ➤ a degree of support from colleagues
> ➤ the individual's personality.

Adapting the five role development stages to a mental health–substance use professional development strategy can offer an additional framework, as an adjunct to a 'capabilities' framework.[22]

By acknowledging the wider dimensions associated with role development (e.g. emotional burden/stress/burn-out/job satisfaction), treatment providers must ensure that these aspects are fundamentally addressed if they seek to attract and retain the 'right people'. Providers must acknowledge the potential emotional demands of role strain and role stress that can be experienced when providing care to individuals with complex needs, experiencing chronic relapsing conditions, or to those who are frequently combative and non-compliant (*see also* Book 2, Chapters 10, 11). This exposure can inevitably lead to stress and psychological morbidity among professionals. For example, a strong association between 'stressors' associated with working in the field of substance use and psychological morbidity.[27] Three categories of stressors identified were alienation, tension and case complexity.[27]

The utility of providing a role development framework for all professionals, alongside the capabilities framework, implicitly acknowledges that technical (knowledge and skill) deficits, or role insecurity, are not of themselves reasons why professionals may be reluctant to engage in mental health–substance use practice. Rather, motivation, attitudes and emotional consideration and relevant organisational support are very important. Figure 10.2 sets out a series of 'role stage scenarios' for mental health–substance use.[22] Professionals, i.e. core, generalist and specialist, could be encouraged, as part of their supervision and ongoing development, to periodically (i.e. every six months) complete a role development inventory for mental health–substance use. This self-assessment tool can provide an opportunity to discuss perceived challenges or barriers to expected transition or progression. Although role development stages are not mapped specifically to the Capabilities levels,[18] it may be expected that 'core' professionals will develop their role up to and including 'engagement', while 'generalist' will need to work towards 'stabilisation' or even 'competency' stages, dependent on their scope of practice.

KEY POINT 10.2

Role development of 'specialists' should cover all five stages.

SUPPORT STRATEGIES

Having assisted the professional to identify their role development stage, specific support strategies can be subsequently explored. A number of training approaches have been employed, ranging from one-off study days, to formalised university level awards. The choice of training required will be variable depending on the capability level and the professional's role development stage. What is recognised is that to ensure that 'training' is embedded into practice it requires the participant being offered the opportunity to 'translate their knowledge to the operational field' and to follow up the training with

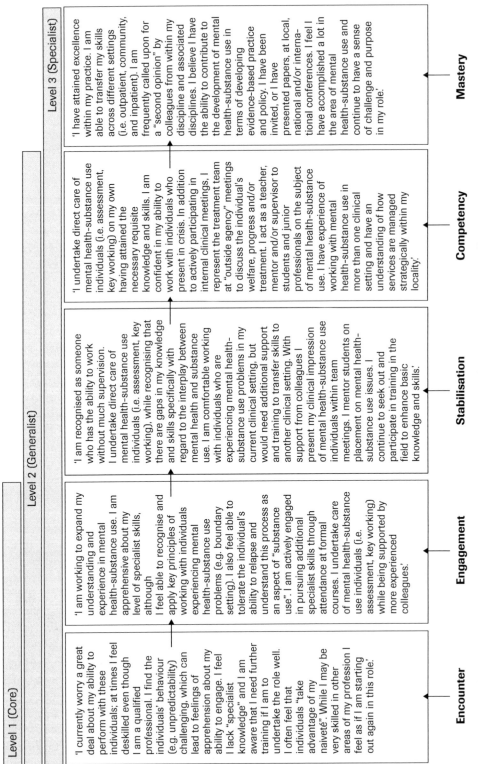

FIGURE 10.2 Role development stage inventory: mental health–substance use practice[22]

Level 1 (Core)

Level 2 (Generalist)

Level 3 (Specialist)

'I currently worry a great deal about my ability to perform with these individuals; at times I feel deskilled even though I am a qualified professional. I find the individuals' behaviour (e.g. unpredictability) challenging, which can lead to feelings of apprehension about my ability to engage. I feel I lack "specialist knowledge" and I am aware that I need further training if I am to undertake the role well. I often feel that individuals "take advantage of my naiveté". While I may be very skilled in other areas of my profession I feel as if I am starting out again in this role.'

'I am working to expand my understanding and experience in mental health–substance use. I am apprehensive about my level of specialist skills, although I feel able to recognise and apply key principles of working with individuals experiencing mental health–substance use problems (e.g. boundary setting). I also feel able to tolerate the individual's ability to relapse and understand this process as an aspect of "substance use". I am actively engaged in pursuing additional specialist skills through attendance at formal courses. I undertake care of mental health–substance use individuals (i.e. assessment, key working) while being supported by more experienced colleagues.'

'I am recognised as someone who has the ability to work without much supervision. I undertake direct care of mental health–substance use individuals (i.e. assessment, key working), while recognising that there are gaps in my knowledge and skills specifically with regard to the interplay between mental health and substance use. I am comfortable working with individuals who are experiencing mental health–substance use problems in my current clinical setting, but would need additional support and training to transfer skills to another clinical setting. With support from colleagues I present my clinical impression of mental health–substance use individuals within team meetings. I mentor students on placement on mental health–substance use issues. I continue to seek out and participate in training in the field to enhance basic knowledge and skills.'

'I undertake direct care of mental health–substance use individuals (i.e. assessment, key working) on my own having attained the necessary requisite knowledge and skills. I am confident in my ability to work with individuals who present in crisis. In addition to actively participating in internal clinical meetings, I represent the treatment team at "outside agency" meetings to discuss the individual's welfare, progress and/or treatment. I act as a teacher, mentor and/or supervisor to students and junior professionals on the subject of mental health–substance use. I have experience of working with mental health–substance use in more than one clinical setting and have an understanding of how services are managed strategically within my locality.'

'I have attained excellence within my practice. I am able to transfer my skills across different settings (i.e. outpatient, community, and inpatient). I am frequently called upon for a "second opinion" by colleagues from within my discipline and associated disciplines. I believe I have the ability to contribute to the development of mental health–substance use in terms of developing evidence-based practice and policy. I have been invited, or I have presented papers, at local, national and/or international conferences. I feel I have accomplished a lot in the area of mental health–substance use and continue to have a sense of challenge and purpose in my role.'

Encounter Engagement Stabilisation Competency Mastery

ongoing supervision support/consultation. Some training programmes have found that the most effective way to train professionals is to integrate training with the day-to-day experience of working together, so that professionals learn from each other in the process. Examples include whole team training, intra- and interdisciplinary training, and the use of an 'expert' to support/supervise/mentor a team.

A more novel initiative with respect to workforce development is the 'Experienced Nurse Job Rotation Scheme'.[28] The model was initially developed to address retention challenges among experienced nursing personnel, who were expressing job dissatisfaction, burn-out, and/or other work-related challenges. In partnership with a local education provider, professionals were sponsored to undertake specific work-based accredited learning, which was undertaken alongside a negotiated rotational work programme offering the opportunity to practise across a number of different clinical areas within the wider organisation. The findings from an evaluation of this scheme indicate a number of positive opportunities/outcomes that have relevance for role development in the area of mental health–substance use. These opportunities are summarised below.

➤ Attainment of accredited training (gaining specific knowledge, skills needed to work with mental health–substance use problems).
➤ Opportunity for participants to change and develop – this particularly was deemed helpful in tackling 'institutionalised practice' (e.g. role legitimacy associated with negative attitudinal legacy towards individuals who use substances). Professionals moving out of their 'comfort zones' increases the possibility for greater self-scrutiny and reflection.
➤ Beneficial impact on fellow professionals, and individuals – participants of the Scheme report a 'transformational role', through the opportunity of being able to undertake more challenges and the chain reaction their 'learning/development' had on their work environments and person-centred care.
➤ Opportunity to merge theory and practice, by simultaneously undertaking accredited training; learning could be operationalised more readily in the field, and embedded.
➤ Job satisfaction – perhaps one of the most important outcomes was the reported increase in job satisfaction, particularly given the links between job satisfaction and job performance, plus the increasing need to 'mainstream' mental health–substance use practice.[28]

CONCLUSION: THE FUTURE PROFESSIONAL

While the focus of this chapter has been on how to enable and empower professionals in relation to their role in mental health–substance use, attention must be given to students who are currently in training. There is an urgent need for treatment providers, service commissioners and educationalists to review how current professionals are being trained with respect to the care and management of the individual with mental health–substance use problems. While greater emphasis is being placed on intra- and interprofessional training/education, there is still a gaping absence of 'fundamental and basic' knowledge and skills in the area of problematic substance use. If there is to be a future mental health–substance use professional 'fit for purpose', a major paradigm shift within current undergraduate training programmes is needed. To conclude, there is a need to address the training and support needs of the individual, and the family. Increasingly, the role and input of the individual and family has been accepted as important in the delivery of services and training of professionals. Consideration on how to best support and incorporate this input into direct training of professionals and students needs to be duly acknowledged, as the 'authentic voice' and 'lived experiences' have enormous impact and credence in facilitating changes in attitudes, stereotype and prejudice.

REFERENCES

1 Skinner N, Feather NT, Freeman T, *et al*. Stigma and discrimination in health care provision to drug users: the role of values, affect and deservingness judgments. *J Appl Socl Psychol*. 2007; **37**: 163–86.

2 National Health Service Confederation. *Seeing Double: meeting the challenge of dual diagnosis*. Briefing Paper. September 2009. Available at: www.nhsconfed.org/publications/briefings/2009-Briefings/Pages/Seeing-double-meeting-challenge.aspx (accessed 16 February 2010).

3 Scottish Executive. 2005. *National Strategy for the Development of the Social Services Professional*. Available at: www.scotland.gov.uk/Publications/2005/11/07104403/44051 (accessed 16 February 2010). p. 1.

4 Skinner N, Roche AM, Freeman T, *et al*. Health professionals' attitudes towards AOD-related work: moving the traditional focus from education and training to organizational culture. *Drugs: education, prevention and policy*. 2009; **16**: 232–49.

5 Department of Health. *Mental Health Policy Implementation Guide: dual diagnosis good practice guide*. London: Department of Health; 2002. Available at: www.dh.gov.uk/en/Publicationsandstatistics/Publications/PublicationsPolicyAndGuidance/DH_4009058 (accessed 16 February 2010). p. 10.

6 Davies A, Huxley P. Survey of general practitioners' opinions on treatment of opiate users. *BMJ*. 1997; **314**: 1173–4.

7 Foster JH, Onyeukwu C. The attitudes of forensic nurses to substance using service users. *J Psychiatr Ment Health Nurs*. 2003; **10**: 578–84.

8 Pinikahana J, Happell B, Carta B. Mental health professionals' attitudes to drugs and substance abuse. *Nurs Health Sci*. 2002; **4**: 57–62.

9 McLaughlin D, Long A. An extended literature review of health professionals' perceptions of illicit drugs and their individuals who use them. *J Psychiatr Ment Health Nurs*. 1996; **3**: 283–8.

10 O'Gara C, Keaney F, Best D, *et al*. Substance misuse training among psychiatric doctors, psychiatric nurses, medical students and nursing students in a South London psychiatric teaching hospital. *Drugs: education, prevention and policy*. 2005; **12**: 327–36.

11 Aanavi MP, Taube DO, Ja DY, *et al*. The status of psychologists' training about and treatment of substance-abusing clients. *J Psychoactive Drugs*. 1999; **31**: 441–4.

12 International Centre for Drug Policy. *Substance Misuse in the Undergraduate Medical Curriculum*. A United Kingdom Medical Schools' collaborative programme. International Centre for Drug Policy (ICDP); 2007. Available at: www.sgul.ac.uk/about-st-georges/divisions/faculty-of-medicine-and-biomedical-sciences/mental-health/icdp/our-work-programmes/substance-misuse-in-the-undergraduate-medical-curriculum-1/substance-misuse-in-the-undergraduate-medical-curriculum/(accessed 23 February 2010).

13 William K. Attitudes of mental health professionals to co-morbidity between mental health problems and substance misuse. *J Ment Health*. 1999; **8**: 605–13.

14 Royal College of Psychiatrists. *Co-existing Problems of Mental Disorder and Substance Misuse (Dual Diagnosis): A training needs analysis*. Technical Report, College Research Unit (CRU). London: Royal College of Psychiatrists; 2001.

15 Sainsbury Centre for Mental Health. *The Capable Practitioner: a framework and list of the practitioner capabilities required to implement the National Service Framework for Mental Health.* The Training & Practice Development Section of the Sainsbury Centre for Mental Health: London; 2001. Available at: www.centreformentalhealth.org.uk/pdfs/the_capable_practitioner.pdf (accessed 2 September 2010). p. 22.

16 Department of Health. *National Service Framework for Mental Health.* London: Department of Health; 1999. Available at: www.dh.gov.uk/en/Publicationsandstatistics/Publications/PublicationsPolicyAndGuidance/DH_4009598 (accessed 16 February 2010).

17 Morrison T. *DANOS: the Drug and Alcohol National Occupational Standards.* Available at: www.alcohol-drugs.co.uk/DANOS/DANOS.html (accessed 16 February 2010).

18 Hughes L. *Closing the Gap: a capability framework for working effectively with people with combined mental health and substance use problems (Dual Diagnosis).* Lincoln: Centre for Clinical and Academic Professional Innovation, University of Lincoln; 2006. Available at: www.lincoln.ac.uk/ccawi/publications/Closing%20the%20Gap.pdf (accessed 16 February 2010).

19 Shaw S, Cartwright A, Spratley T, *et al. Responding to Drinking Problems.* London: Croom Helm; 1978.

20 WordNet Search 3. s.v. 'role'. Available at: http://wordnetweb.princeton.edu/perl/webwn (accessed 16 February 2010).

21 Biddle BJ. *Role Theory: expectations, identities, and behaviors.* New York, NY: Academic Press; 1979. p. 8.

22 Clancy C, Oyefeso A, Ghodse H. Role development and career stages in addiction nursing: an exploratory study. *J Adv Nurs.* 2007; **57**: 161–71.

23 Brookes K, Davidson PM, Daly J, *et al.* Role theory: a framework to investigate the community nurse role in contemporary health care systems. *Contemp Nurse.* 2007; **25**: 146–55.

24 Farnell S, Dawson D. 'It's not like the wards'. Experiences of nurses new to critical care: a qualitative study. *Int J Nurs Stud.* 2006; **43**: 319–31.

25 Rosser M, King L. Transition experiences of qualified nurses moving into hospice nursing. *J Adv Nurs.* 2003; **43**: 206–15.

26 Brown MA, Olshansky EF. From limbo to legitimacy: a theoretical model of the transition to the primary care nurse practitioner role. *Nurs Res.* 1997; **48**: 46–51.

27 Oyefeso A, Clancy C, Farmer R. Prevalence and associated factors in burn-out and psychological morbidity among substance misuse professionals. *BMC Health Serv Res.* 2008; **8**: 39.

28 Lucock R, Coyne P. *Experienced Nurse Job Rotation Scheme: phase two final evaluation.* London: Central and North West London Mental Health NHS Trust; 2006. Available at: www.nurserotation.com/ExpNurseTwo.htm (accessed 16 February 2010).

TO LEARN MORE

A briefing report from the National Mental Health Development Unit (the NHS Confederation) on dual diagnosis workforce issues. Available at: www.nmhdu.org.uk/silo/files/seeing-double-meeting-the-challenge-of-dual-diagnosis.pdf

Australia's National Research Centre on AOD Workforce Development. Available at: www.nceta.flinders.edu.au

Closing the Gap Capabilities Framework. Available at: www.lincoln.ac.uk/ccawi/publications/Closing%20the%20Gap.pdf

Dual Diagnosis Toolkits – Training Frontline Staff. Available at: http://download.ncadi.samhsa.gov/ken/pdf/toolkits/cooccurring/EBPKIT_CoOccur_Training.pdf

Nurse Rotation. Available at: www.nurserotation.com

CHAPTER 11

Attitudes and brief training interventions: a practical approach

Philip D Cooper

INTRODUCTION

There is an identified need to improve the standards of service delivery for people with mental health–substance use problems, and ensure care provision is equitable and consistent at all points of access into, and through, services. To effectively meet the needs of people with mental health–substance use problems, services should aim to promote an ethos of care based in recovery and harm reduction approaches, and foster a 'no wrong door' whole systems integrated approach to care delivery. To achieve this, and successfully move towards a whole systems integrated approach to care, it is essential that all professionals (*unqualified and qualified*), have the knowledge and skills to provide effective, timely, evidence-based interventions, and support people in making informed decisions about their substance use. Moreover, professionals must feel confident and supported in providing these interventions.

This chapter considers the impact of professionals' attitudes on care provision for people who experience mental health–substance use problems and how brief training interventions may improve the professionals' knowledge, skills and confidence, and promote positive attitudes. The chapter outlines the steps required to provide an effective training programme, which meets the needs of the professional, and, most importantly, meets the needs of people experiencing mental health–substance use problems. The chapter demonstrates how this has been achieved within the author's work environment.

SELF-ASSESSMENT EXERCISE 11.1

> **Time: 15 minutes**
> Consider your workplace.
> - How does your service/team currently support people with mental health–substance use problems?
> - What support is available to you to assist in this?
> - What training is currently available in your trust/organisation/local area to help you improve your knowledge and skills?

WORKFORCE CAPABILITIES AND PROFESSIONAL ATTITUDES

A major issue in relation to delivering integrated care for mental health–substance use problems is the concern that professionals significantly lack the knowledge and skills to adequately meet the needs of people with mental health–substance use problems. One key barrier to providing effective care management and interventions arises from a lack of understanding, and inadequate preparation in pre- and post-registration training. Pre-registration substance use training for medical, nursing and social work professionals has been found to be unacceptably low in comparison to its prevalence,[1-3] and post-registration training for mental health–substance use problems has not been considered a priority.[4] Where training is available, the relevance and quality is important to consider. Substance use training for professionals is often considered in isolation with pre-registration training tending to focus only on the physical identification of substances and their pharmacological effects.[5] Unfortunately, post-registration training offers little in the way of developing this baseline knowledge and skills.

SELF-ASSESSMENT EXERCISE 11.2

Time: 15 minutes
- How much training did you receive pre-/post-registration?
- How well do you think this training prepared you to work with people with mental health–substance use problems?
- How confident did/do you feel in supporting people with mental health–substance use problems?
- Do you think the above affected your interactions with people with mental health–substance use problems? If so, how?

Professional attitudes and commitment to working with substance-using individuals are influenced by their perceptions of:
➤ **role adequacy**: a perceived lack of knowledge and skill in identifying and responding to substance-using individuals
➤ **role legitimacy**: uncertainty as to whether, or how far, harmful substance use falls within their remit
➤ **role support**: insufficient access or support from specialist services/professionals, should they identify a harmful substance user (*see* Chapter 10).[6]

A triad of knowledge and skill acquisition, appropriate support and clinical experience were perceived as integral components in ensuring *role security* and *high therapeutic commitment*. Where the professional experienced role security and high therapeutic commitment, positive attitudes prevailed.[6] Therefore, the professional with positive therapeutic attitudes are more likely to accurately identify, and confidently respond to, substance use problems, thus improving individual outcomes.[6] It is now widely recognised that professionals' perceptions of these concepts directly affect their response to substance-using individuals.[4,7,8]

SELF-ASSESSMENT EXERCISE 11.3

> **Time: 15 minutes**
> - Within the context of your role, what knowledge, skills and attitudes do you need to achieve *role security* and *high therapeutic commitment*?
> - What could result if you experienced *role insecurity*?

DIFFICULT TO ENGAGE INDIVIDUALS OR DIFFICULT TO ENGAGE PROFESSIONALS? THE CYCLE OF DISENGAGEMENT

Engaging people in services by developing therapeutic and mutually trusting relationships is an essential first step in providing effective interventions. Without a period of positive engagement, subsequent interventions are unlikely to be successful. Professional attitudes are a significant determinant in the engagement process and in the development of therapeutic relationships. Where negative attitudes exist, the quality of care and treatment outcomes for people with mental health–substance use problems are reduced,[9,10] and mutually respecting and trusting relationships are unlikely to thrive (*see also* Book 3, Chapter 3; Book 5, Chapter 7).

People who use substances are often viewed as unmotivated, manipulative and self-destructive,[11] and professionals may find it difficult to work with someone perceived as demanding. Such negative perceptions and stereotyping attitudes may result in responses and interactions distinguished by suspicion, mistrust and avoidance from both parties.[12]

When the professionals' perceptions of *role adequacy, legitimacy* and *support* are low, they experience *role insecurity*[6] and, consequently, fail to accurately identify and respond to substance users when they experience uncertainty regarding these three concepts. *Role insecurity* derives from inadequate training and/or unsupportive working environments, and is likely to result in professionals feeling intellectually and emotionally unprepared to address substance use problems. Feelings of professional inadequacy may arise, and, subsequently, it becomes beneficial for the professional to fail to recognise and respond to substance users in an attempt to protect their own professional self-esteem. Such threats to professional self-esteem result in safeguarding responses and the countertransference of anxieties to the individual. Consequently, the individual is perceived as unmotivated – therefore, unworthy of the professional's skills. This emotional expression of role insecurity is described as *low therapeutic commitment*.[6] Where therapeutic commitment is low, negative attitudes towards the individual tend to be high, and professionals often disinvest in those people they perceive as unmotivated or are unable/unwilling to engage with the service and treatment offered. When considered from this perspective disengagement may be viewed as being professional-led, as opposed to individual-led (*see* Book 4, Chapter 2).

Individual disengagement can occur for a number of reasons but the role professionals may play in this process cannot be underestimated. It is important for the professional to be aware of their own values, attitudes and beliefs towards people experiencing mental health–substance use problems, and understand how these may impact on the development of therapeutic relationships and treatment outcomes. Awareness of these issues, and how they impact on their interactions with the individual, will enable the professional to become emotionally available, and therapeutically engaged, with people experiencing mental health–substance use problems.[13] Increasing the professionals' understanding of mental health–substance use problems, improving their knowledge, skills and confidence, and challenging negative attitudes by providing ongoing and progressive training, can be a valuable first step in reducing some of the traditional barriers people experience in accessing the support they need.

SELF-ASSESSMENT EXERCISE 11.4

> **Time: 10 minutes**
> Explore your feelings and views towards the individual with mental health–substance use problems. If you have not experienced this situation first hand, visualise a potential scenario where you are the professional providing care.
> • Make notes of your feelings.
> • How do you think your feelings and views may affect your therapeutic relationship with the person you are supporting?

HOW EFFECTIVE ARE BRIEF TRAINING INTERVENTIONS?

Studies have shown that brief training interventions, for non-specialist professionals, can challenge and reduce negative attitudes and improve professional knowledge, skills and confidence in working with people with mental health–substance use problems.[14–16] However, there are three common problems that may reduce the overall effectiveness of brief training initiatives:

1 Non-attendees
2 Post-training support
3 Retention of knowledge/skills.

1 Non-attendees

Where training is not a mandatory requirement it is often only accessed by those with a specific interest. Therefore, non-attendees may consider mental health–substance use problems as less important. Consequently, the possibility of non-attendees holding less favourable attitudes arises, a factor that can limit the overall effectiveness of training initiatives. It has been noted that doctors in training are influenced by the prejudicial attitudes of senior colleagues, tending to ignore what they had been taught in class in favour of these attitudes.[10] Therefore, positive attitudes may be diluted on returning to practice. This problem may also arise where training is mandatory yet not delivered to the whole team, i.e. individual team members attend training at differing times, rather than training being delivered to all team members simultaneously. Although all team members will eventually receive training, this may take a number of years, depending on the frequency of training delivery and size of the organisation. This delay increases the risk of positive changes being diluted on return to practice in favour of existing and dominant attitudes and sub-therapeutic clinical practices.

SELF-ASSESSMENT EXERCISE 11.5

Time: 15 minutes
You are a practice educator and trainer in your trust/organisation or a clinical lead for mental health–substance use in your work environment. How might you overcome the many and varied opinions and approaches of the professional team to positively change existing negative attitudes/behaviours?

2 Post-training support

If senior colleagues hold less positive attitudes and do not embrace positive changes in practice, attendees may not feel fully supported on returning to the clinical environment. Ongoing support and supervision is essential in any training initiative and the long-term efficacy of training interventions may be diminished without adequate post-training support. Role support is identified as a key aspect in developing and maintaining therapeutic attitudes.[6] Providing post-training support and supervision enables the embedding of new skills and practices and improve the overall aims of training initiatives.

SELF-ASSESSMENT EXERCISE 11.6

Time: 30 minutes
Review current practice in your work environment.
- Is regular clinical supervision supported and encouraged?
- What other forms of support exist within your work environment, trust, or organisation?
- If so, how does this benefit your practice?
- How does it enhance and improve empirical and aesthetic knowledge?

3 Retention of knowledge/skills

While there are numerous recommendations on training content, and increasing evidence to support the use of training in challenging negative attitudes and increasing knowledge and skills, there is limited evidence to suggest these recommendations and training initiatives have the desired effect in the long term. The efficacy of short, isolated educational courses on the attitudes of the professional has been questioned, and the need to examine how the design and frequency of such courses can be improved to meet their aims has been identified.[12] Without the provision of refresher sessions, and opportunities to develop knowledge and skills over time, organisations will find it difficult to move towards integrated approaches to care and ensure the workforce (professionals qualified and unqualified) are adequately equipped to address the needs of people with mental health–substance use problems.

Overcoming these issues

Adopting a whole team approach to training enables each professional to be more responsive in addressing the needs of individuals, and provides a foundation from which adequate peer support networks may be developed. In addition, it enables discussions that are relevant to that specific clinical area and assists the team to identify unified and consistent approaches to care.

To provide sustainable and effective training programmes, which aim to fully prepare each professional to respond to, and address, mental health–substance use problems, it is necessary to view training as *more than* a 'one-off' taught event. Training must be an ongoing developmental process that adopts a number of approaches to achieve the desired outcomes. It must be progressive to enable the development of knowledge and skills in the long term. This leads to a workforce that is increasingly enabled to respond to mental health–substance use problems, and fosters the notion that working with the individual experiencing mental health–substance use problems is part of the organisa- tion's 'core business'. In addition, the efficacy of training initiatives on professionals' knowledge, skills and confidence must be evaluated, as must the duration of training effects so that the frequency of refresher courses can be set to maintain classroom gains. Ensuring adequate peer support networks, intra- and interdisciplinary, are available at all levels is an essential element in this process of sustained change, and will increase the likelihood of training initiatives achieving the desired outcome.

The importance of a multifaceted approach, rather than one single route, to improv- ing the practitioner capabilities cannot be overemphasised.[17] A number of pivotal development points have been recommended to achieve this:

➤ Training that engenders networking and integrated care pathways across organisational boundaries.
➤ Developing protocols with higher education providers that identify work-based learning opportunities.
➤ Developing regional support networks that promote open learning and shared opportunities to explore positive clinical work in [mental health–substance use].
➤ Work rotation secondments.
➤ Partnership commissioning and ownership of [mental health–substance use] posts.
➤ Developing across-service level agreements to share learning opportunities.
➤ Developing an electronic web-based learning package and toolkit on [mental health–substance use].[17]

DEVELOPING TRAINING AT A LOCAL LEVEL
To provide brief training initiatives that are effective and sustainable, a 'four-step' approach is required prior to the delivery of training sessions:

Step 1: Undertake a training needs analysis
Step 2: Develop a training strategy
Step 3: Training design
Step 4: Implement training.

A fifth step should be added post education and training:
Step 5: Evaluate the effectiveness of training.

Step 1: Training needs analysis

An essential precursor to the development and delivery of any training initiative is the undertaking of a training needs analysis to understand the specific needs of each professional within the organisation/service(s), and identify strengths and deficits in addressing mental health–substance use problems. Co-opting a small and focused working group can be beneficial at this stage. Ideally, the group should continue to exist throughout the lifetime of the project. Membership should include one or more:

➤ individual(s) who have experienced mental health–substance use problems
➤ member(s) of the family or carer(s)
➤ professional(s) representing mental health services
➤ professional(s) representing substance use services
➤ professional(s) representing non-statutory services.

A working group can provide a wealth of knowledge, experience and views that will be invaluable in developing an effective training programme. In addition, tasks can be shared between group members so that one person is not unnecessarily overburdened.

In carrying out a training needs analysis, the working group will need to do the following.

➤ Identify training needs of each professional (qualified or unqualified).
➤ Consider the training needs of each clinical area – although all professionals will require shared baseline knowledge and skill sets (e.g. knowledge of commonly used substances; skills in screening and assessment), the needs of inpatient versus assertive outreach professionals may differ significantly, with the latter requiring more training in long-term interventions and strategies, and the former brief interventions. Similarly, substance use professionals will require less training around substance use than their colleagues in mental health settings, but will require more on identifying and addressing mental health problems.
➤ Consider the training needs of individual posts within teams – again, while all professionals (qualified or unqualified) should share common knowledge and skills, particularly in identifying problems and providing brief interventions, qualified professionals are expected to carry out more thorough assessments and complex interventions.

A useful tool to identify professionals' knowledge, skills and confidence is the Comorbidity Problems Perceptions Questionnaire.[18] This tool measures therapeutic attitudes and role competency of non-specialist professionals working with people who experience mental health–substance use problems. It is an adaptation of the Alcohol and Alcohol Problems Perceptions Questionnaire,[6] and the Drug and Drug Problems Perceptions Questionnaire,[18] and specifically considers the professionals' therapeutic attitudes in relation to the concepts of role adequacy, role legitimacy and role support. The Comorbidity Problems Perceptions Questionnaire is a 33-item questionnaire and respondents are invited to indicate the strength of their agreement to a given statement on a scale from 1 (strongly agree), to 7 (strongly disagree). A high total score indicates poor therapeutic attitudes and a low score, positive therapeutic attitudes. In addition to identifying training needs, this tool is a useful for evaluating the efficacy of training initiatives by allowing a comparison of pre- and post-training scores.

Step 2: Develop a training strategy

The findings of the training needs analysis should inform the development of a training strategy, which should be incorporated into a wider strategy highlighting how mental health–substance use problems are addressed locally. The training strategy should identify the professionals' strengths and deficits and outline a training plan to address these. It should:

➤ highlight the professionals' responsibilities to access training
➤ indicate who should receive training, and at what level
➤ identify any priority areas for training delivery.

In developing the training strategy the working group should undertake a review of existing training provision to ensure:

➤ it meets local needs and is relevant to the local population
➤ it meets the needs of differing clinical areas and professionals within those areas
➤ its content is based on national policy and guidelines, and best practice guidance
➤ it addresses concepts of role legitimacy, role adequacy and role support
➤ it is progressive and enables the development of knowledge and skills over time.

Step 3: Training design

If a current training provision does not fully address the issues outlined above it will be necessary to redesign existing training or develop new training packages. It can be useful to evaluate the content and efficacy of training from other areas to consider their relevance to locally assessed need. If training packages available in the public domain meet local need it may not be necessary to develop training from scratch. Two examples of publicly available training packages are as follows.

1 *Ten Essential Shared Capabilities Advanced Module: combined mental health and substance use problems (dual diagnosis).*[19] Aimed primarily at mental health professionals, the package comprises 16 modules covering drug and alcohol awareness, assessment, treatment and relapse prevention. Didactic teaching is minimal and learning is mainly facilitated by group exercises and role play. Resources include a training manual, PowerPoint presentations, trainer's resources, and additional materials. The complete training package is available for download at: www.lincoln. ac.uk/ccawi/ESC-DD.html.

2 *PsyCheck.*[20] Aimed primarily at substance use professionals, PsyCheck offers a validated screening tool for mental health problems in substance users and an evidence-based treatment intervention. Training can be delivered over four half or two full days and develops attendees' skills in the use of the PsyCheck screening tool and in delivering a cognitive behavioural-based intervention. An online version of the training is also available. Resources include: a screening tool users guide; clinical treatment guideline; training and clinical supervision guidelines; programme implementation guidelines; training slides; and training resources. The complete training package can be downloaded from: www.psycheck.org.au/index.html.

If it is necessary to develop new training packages to fully meet local needs, the 'Dual Diagnosis Capabilities Framework'[8] is extremely useful to benchmark training against. This framework identifies 19 capabilities across three sections (*Values, Utilising*

Knowledge and Skills, and *Practice Development*) and three differing levels of competence (*Core, Generalist,* and *Specialist*), which assists in identifying the knowledge and skill requirements of specific professional groups. The content of training should be based on relevant national policy/recommendations and reflect the needs of the local community. Decisions on how training is best delivered locally (e.g. whole team training or other), its duration and frequency, and whether one, or a number of, levels of training are required to fully meet the needs of the workforce will need to be considered.

In addition to developing a training package, an effective model of peer support and supervision needs to be identified to embed new skills in practice and maintain knowledge and skill gains in the long term. Such a model may involve the identification of link professionals in each clinical area. Ideally, link professionals will receive additional training and their role should include:

➤ developing effective working relationships with substance use–mental health teams to facilitate joint working, and offer support and advice where required
➤ arranging joint assessments, where required
➤ acting as a resource to fellow professionals in the implementation of new practices.

It is essential that link professionals receive ongoing support and supervision, which could be achieved through the initiation of peer support and educational forums.

Step 4: Implement training

Prior to rolling out training to the whole organisation it may be beneficial to pilot training. This will enable an evaluation of the content and allow changes to be made to either individual sessions or the structure of session delivery. In addition, it will enable an evaluation of the effectiveness of training on professionals' knowledge, skills, confidence and attitudes by assessing these areas before and after training. Once the pilot has been completed, and the necessary adjustments made, the training can be delivered across the organisation. Teams with the highest level of need and contact with people with mental health–substance use problems should take priority. These teams should have been identified in the training needs analysis.

Step 5: Evaluate the effectiveness of training

Initiatives aimed at improving service delivery require constant monitoring and assessment to measure efficacy. Measurements for improvement are linked to strategy aims and objectives and assist in demonstrating whether changes are making the desired improvements.[21] The 'Model for Improvement' and the 'Plan, Do, Study, Act cycle'[22] provide useful tools for measuring improvement and their use should be ongoing.

The Comorbidity Problems Perceptions Questionnaire[18] is useful for monitoring and evaluating improvement in the professionals' knowledge, skills and attitudes. Considering the long-term effect of training on these areas is important and may assist in identifying the required frequency of 'refresher' and further training.

The impact of training on the standard of care provided, and intervention/treatment outcomes, is fundamentally important and the experience of the individual and family in evaluation is essential. The UK Modernisation Agency[23] advocates the use of focus groups, individual diaries, and discovery interviews to facilitate this end. The individual and family representatives should maintain a presence in the working group throughout the project's lifespan, preferable through membership, or at least, consultation.

A final area of consideration is benchmarking. Evaluating the outcomes of a training programme against existing, proven training initiatives will be beneficial.

BRIEF TRAINING IN PRACTICE

This section provides an example of how Suffolk Mental Health Partnership National Health Service Trust has responded to the issues outlined. To address the needs of people experiencing mental health–substance use problems, and ensure professionals feel confident and supported in providing care to this group, the Trust has adopted a three-tiered 'training and support model' to provide the foundations of a move towards an integrated model of care. The three tiers of training are outlined below, in addition to other initiatives to support this.

Level 1: Mandatory baseline training

This two-day mandatory training is for all professionals (qualified and unqualified), who are likely to be in contact with people experiencing mental health–substance use problems. Due to the differing needs of the professional in mental health and substance use services, two courses are available: one for mental health professionals; one for substance use professionals. The mental health professionals' course is outlined below.

The baseline training for mental health professionals was designed to address the concepts of role adequacy and role legitimacy, and its content based on report recommendations.[24–7] In addition, the content has been mapped against the Dual Diagnosis Capability Framework.[8]

Day 1 consists of six taught hours, and aims to:

➤ develop knowledge and understanding of the complex needs of people with mental health–substance use problems

➤ recognise the challenges faced by services, the professional, the individual and the family in providing and accessing support/services

➤ understand the mutually dependent and complex nature of a person's mental health and substance use

➤ develop knowledge on commonly used substances and the potential effects on a person's physical, psychological and social well-being

➤ encourage participants to reflect on their own values, attitudes and beliefs toward people who use substances.

Day 2 consists of six taught hours, and commences with a presentation from the local substance use team. This session aims to provide participants with a clearer understanding of the role and function of the substance use service and dispel any unrealistic expectations held by mental health professionals on what the service is commissioned to provide. An important aspect of this session is to introduce participants to the four-tiered approach to drug treatment in the UK,[28] and highlight the role non-specialist professionals have in providing interventions to people who use substances.

The second session focuses on increasing participants' understanding of the nature of behaviour change. Ensuring the professional understands the process of change, and the difficulties people encounter in changing behaviour, is essential. Professionals can often become frustrated, unsupportive and dismissive of individuals' repeated change attempts, and place unrealistic expectations on individuals to change on the first or second attempt (*see* Book 4, Chapter 6). To challenge these expectations participants are asked to reflect, in pairs, on a time when they attempted to change behaviour (e.g. dieting, smoking cessation, a new exercise regime, etc.) and consider the difficulties they experienced in maintaining positive changes.

The remainder of the day focuses on developing participants' skills in screening for substance use problems using the Alcohol, Drugs, and Substance Involvement Screening Test[29] (commonly referred to as ASSIST), assessment of substance use, and brief interventions. Table 11.1 outlines the content of the two study days.

TABLE 11.1 Level 1: Baseline mental health–substance use problems training for mental health professionals

Day 1	Day 2
1 *Mental health–substance use*: definition and challenges	1 The role of substance use treatment services and local services
2 Alcohol and mental health	2 The Cycle of Change and Four Stage Model
3 Cannabis and mental health	3 Essentials of assessment
4 Stimulants and mental health	4 Substance use screening and screening tools
5 Attitudes and feelings	5 Brief intervention.
6 Legal issues.	

Level 2: Intermediate training

Intermediate training is for all qualified professionals working with people experiencing mental health–substance use problems and aims to increase participants' knowledge and skills in working with people in the long term. The course utilises the Four Stage Model[30] as a framework for content delivery (Engagement, Motivation, Active Treatment and Relapse Prevention – *see* Book 4, Chapter 7; Book 5, Chapters 7, 11; Book 6, Chapters 15, 16), and is mapped against the Dual Diagnosis Capability Framework.[8] This training is mandatory for link professionals from each clinical area, in addition to being accessible to those who wish to further develop their knowledge and skills. Participants must have completed the baseline training prior to undertaking this level.

This level comprises four days' training, split into two sets of two days, with a three month gap between. Participants are usually a mix of mental health and substance use professionals, which aims to encourage the sharing of knowledge and skills, leading towards the fostering of positive working relationships. In addition to the taught elements, the course adopts an 'action learning' approach. Action learning is an educational process where participants 'learn by doing' and study their own actions and experience with the aim of improving future performance. The action learning element of the course takes place between the two sets of two days and participants are given 7.5 hours protected time away from the workplace to undertake this. Participants are encouraged to work in pairs or small groups, preferably with participants from differing service areas, on a particular case or service issue. Each is encouraged to utilise the knowledge and skills they have gained in the baseline training and the first two days of the intermediate course, in addition to existing skills. This approach aims to serve a number of purposes. It:

➤ continues learning beyond the classroom and for a period of three months, as opposed to four days
➤ encourages reflection on past/current approaches to mental health–substance use problems
➤ increases participants' confidence in addressing mental health–substance use problems
➤ improves participants' understanding of the role and function of other services
➤ increases the effectiveness of joint working between teams/services by developing good working relationships
➤ improves individual and service outcomes by the sharing and pooling of knowledge and skills.

Facilitator support is available to participants throughout if required. Participants feed back to the group at the start of day three, and group discussion enables further reflection on practice and the possible identification of alternative approaches and future action points. Table 11.2 outlines the content of the four study days.

TABLE 11.2 Level 2: Intermediate mental health–substance use problems training

Days 1 and 2	Days 3 and 4
1 Engaging people with mental health–substance use problems	1 Action learning groups – feedback and discussion
2 Effective care coordination for individuals with complex needs	2 Recovery in mental health–substance use
3 Action learning groups	3 Harm reduction approaches
4 Motivational interviewing and mental health–substance use problems	4 Medication management
5 Cognitive behaviour therapy and mental health–substance use problems.	5 Relapse prevention and early warning signs monitoring
	6 Family interventions.

Level 3: Advanced training
Level 3 training is available for professionals who want to develop advanced skills in working with people with mental health–substance use problems and attain accreditation. These courses are available from external institutions and can be achieved via a number of methods. For example, Middlesex University, London, UK, offer a range of accredited courses in mental health–substance use problems, from Advanced Diploma level through to Master of Science, which can be studied by attendance or via distance learning (*see* www.mdx.ac.uk/courses/postgraduate/nursing_midwifery_health/).

OTHER INITIATIVES TO SUPPORT LEARNING
Mental health–substance use problems clinical resource packs have been developed

in recognition of a lack of accurate information available at clinical level. Two packs are available for:
1 mental health professionals
2 substance use professionals.

Developed within Suffolk, both packs highlight the key issues for the individual experiencing mental health–substance use problems, provide information on commonly used substances, mental health problems and a range of interventions that may be useful in the treatment of mental health–substance use problems. The packs act as an accompaniment to training and contain screening tools introduced in the training. However, the packs only provide a brief overview and simply act as a point of reference for additional information.

In addition to the packs, a mental health–substance use problems e-list interest group has developed within the Suffolk Trust. With current membership of over 120 professional members, the e-list encourages the exchange and distribution of up-to-date information (e.g. news, reports, published papers, etc.) relating to mental health–substance use problems between list members with the aim of increasing knowledge and keeping list members up to date with the latest developments.

A final initiative is the development of a mental health–substance use problems operational forum. Forums are held quarterly and a representative from each clinical area/team across the county (Suffolk) is invited to attend, in addition to partner agencies and the individual who has experienced mental health–substance use services. The forum aims to provide:

➤ regular updates on local developments
➤ an opportunity for mental health and substance use professionals, statutory and non-statutory, to discuss complex issues and develop working relationships
➤ an opportunity to develop knowledge through educational sessions
➤ an opportunity to develop a deeper understanding of the role of different teams and routes of referral for these teams
➤ ongoing support to link professionals
➤ an opportunity to be involved in service development by consultation and working group initiatives
➤ a link between the clinical area and the Trust's mental health–substance use problems steering group.

CONCLUSION
While in the early stages of transition and developments this chapter provides examples of how an organisation may start to move towards ensuring the workforce is adequately prepared to meet the needs of people with mental health–substance use problems, and that people experiencing these problems feel valued and supported in making the changes they feel are important. This training and support model can be achieved with limited cost implications for the organisation but maximum benefit for all involved. The efficacy of this approach, in conjunction with other strategic initiatives, will be monitored and reported on as the project develops.

Effective clinical care necessitates a positive attitude towards people with mental health–substance use problems, and an adequate knowledge base,[10] and training has an unequivocal function in developing positive attitudes among professionals. For positive attitudes to prevail, professionals must be empowered to effectively and confidently:

➤ assess the individual's needs
➤ provide timely interventions and treatment
➤ activate defined and appropriate care pathways.

To fully overcome the barriers people face in accessing services and ensure that care provision is equitable and consistent at all points into and through services, mental health–substance use problems training must be incorporated into pre- and post-registration curriculum. The provision of training in substance use alone without consideration for the mutually dependent and influencing aspects of mental health and substance use is insufficient. To effect a positive change in attitudes and practice, training must be:

➤ progressive
➤ cognisant of the complex needs of the individual with mental health–substance use problems
➤ incorporate a synthesis of didactic and experiential teaching methods
➤ be relevant to the professionals' clinical area.

Moreover, networks of support must be established to facilitate the development of knowledge, embed new skills in practice, and maintain therapeutic attitudes.

The move towards a whole systems integrated approach to care delivery is both difficult and challenging. To successfully achieve this it is essential that services invest in developing the professionals' knowledge and skills, and support them in making positive changes to practice. Without this, it is unlikely that people who experience mental health–substance use problems will receive the high quality standard of care we all expect from the professionals who help the individual make positive changes in their lives.

> Just as a diamond can only be polished by another diamond, it is only through genuine all out engagement with others that people can polish their character, and help each other to reach greater heights.[31]

KEY POINTS 11.1

1 All mental healthcare and substance use professionals should:
- have a good knowledge and understanding of the effects of alcohol and other drugs
- understand the mutually dependent nature of mental health and substance use problems
- be able to screen and assess for mental health and substance use problems
- be able to provide a brief intervention for such problems.
2 Training should:
- start at pre-registration level
- be progressive and aim to build knowledge, skills and confidence in working with mental health–substance use problems in the long term.

3 Whole team training should be considered where possible.

4 Adequate support systems need to be in place to support professionals, and maintain/develop classroom gains.

5 Long-term efficacy of brief training interventions needs to be considered, and the frequency and nature of updates should be established.

6 The effect of training on professionals' attitudes, confidence, knowledge and skills needs to be evaluated and training adjusted to ensure positive changes are achieved and maintained.

7 Most importantly, does training and changes in attitudes and practice have a positive effect on the individual's outcomes?

REFERENCES

1 Crome IB. The trouble with training: substance misuse education in British medical schools revisited. What are the issues? *Drugs: Educ Prev Pol.* 1999; **6**: 111–23.

2 Crome IB, Shaikh N. Undergraduate medical school education in substance misuse in Britain III: can medical students drive change? *Drugs: Educ Prev Pol.* 2004; **11**(6): 483–503.

3 Galvani S, Forrester D. *What Works in Training Social Professionals about Drug and Alcohol Use? A survey of student learning and readiness to practice.* Final Report October 2008. University of Bedfordshire; 2008. Available at: www.beds.ac.uk/departments/appliedsocialstudies/staff/sarah-galvani/galvani-forrester-horeport2008pdf (accessed 17 February 2010).

4 Mears A, Clancy C, Banerjee S, *et al. Co-existing Problems of Mental Disorder and Substance Misuse ('Dual Diagnosis'): a training needs analysis.* London: Royal College of Psychiatrists Research Unit; 2001.

5 Rassool H. Professional education and training. In: Rassool H, Gafoor M, editors. *Addiction Nursing: perspectives on professional and clinical practice.* Cheltenham: Stanley Thorne Ltd; 1997.

6 Shaw S, Cartwright A, Spratley T, *et al. Responding to Drinking Problems.* London: Croom Helm; 1978.

7 Billingham J. Substance misuse education in social work practice. *J Subst Use.* 1999; **4**: 76–81.

8 Hughes L. *Closing the Gap: a capability framework for working effectively with people with combined mental health and substance use problems.* Lincoln: Centre for Clinical and Academic Professional Innovation; 2006. Available at: www.lincoln.ac.uk/ccawi/publications/Closing%20the%20Gap.pdf (accessed 17 February 2010).

9 Foster JH, Onyeukwu C. The attitudes of forensic nurses to substance using people. *J Psychiatr Ment Health Nurs.* 2003; **10**: 578–84.

10 Renner JA Jnr. How to train residents to identify and treat dual diagnosis patients. *Biol Psychiatry.* 2004; **56**: 810–16.

11 Banerjee J, Clancy C, Crome I. *Co-existing Problems of Mental Disorder and Substance Misuse ('Dual Diagnosis'): an information manual 2002.* London: Royal College of Psychiatrists Research Unit; 2002.

12 Richmond IC, Foster JH. Negative attitudes towards people with co-morbid mental health and substance misuse problems: an investigation of mental health professionals. *J Ment Health.* 2003; **12**: 393–403.

13 Cooper PD. The person who experiences mental health and substance use problems. In: Barker, P, editor. *Psychiatric and Mental Health Nursing: the craft of caring.* 2nd ed. London: Hodder Arnold; 2009.

14 Munro A, Watson HE, McFadyen A. Assessing the impact of training on mental health nurses'

therapeutic attitudes and knowledge about co-morbidity: a randomised control trial. *Int J Nurs Stud.* 2007; **44**: 1430–8.

15 Hughes E. A pilot study of dual diagnosis training in prisons. *J Ment Health Prof Dev.* 2006; **1**: 5–14.

16 Hughes E, Wanigarante S, Gourney K, *et al.* Training in dual diagnosis interventions (the COMO study): a randomised control trial. *BMC Psychiatry* . 2008; **8**: 12. Available at: www.biomedcentral.com/1471–244X/8/12 (accessed 17 February 2010).

17 Care Services Improvement Partnership. *Dual Diagnosis: developing capable professionals to improve services and increase positive individual experience.* London: Care Services Improvement Partnership; 2008.

18 Watson H, Maclaren W, Shaw F, *et al. Measuring Professional Attitudes to People with Drug Problems: the development of a tool.* Edinburgh: Effective Interventions Unit, Scottish Executive Drug Misuse Research Programme; 2003.

19 Centre for Clinical and Academic Professional Innovation. *Ten Essential Shared Capabilities Advanced Module: combined mental health and substance use problems (dual diagnosis).* Available at: www.lincoln.ac.uk/ccawi/ESC-DD.htm (accessed 17 February 2010).

20 Lee N, Jenner L, Kay-Lambkin F, *et al. PsyCheck: responding to mental health issues within alcohol and drug treatment.* Canberra, ACT: Commonwealth of Australia; 2007.

21 Modernisation Agency. *Improvement Leaders' Guide: measurement for improvement. Process and systems thinking.* London: Department of Health; 2005.

22 Langley G, Nolan K, Nolan T, *et al. The Improvement Guide: a practical approach to enhancing organizational performance.* San Francisco, CA: Jossey-Bass; 1996.

23 Modernisation Agency. *Improvement Leaders' Guide: involving patients and carers. General improvement skills.* London: Department of Health; 2005.

24 Department of Health. *Mental Health Policy Implementation Guide: dual diagnosis good practice guide.* London: Department of Health; 2002.

25 Department of Health. *Dual Diagnosis in Mental Health Inpatient and Day Hospital Settings: guidance on the assessment and management of patients in mental health inpatient and day hospital settings who have mental ill health and substance use problems.* London: Department of Health; 2006.

26 Department of Health. *The Ten Essential Shared Capabilities: a framework for the whole of the mental health workforce.* London: Department of Health; 2004.

27 Health Advisory Service. *Substance Misuse and Mental Health Comorbidity (Dual Diagnosis): standards for mental health services.* London: Health Advisory Service; 2001.

28 National Treatment Agency for Substance Misuse. *Models of Care for the Treatment of Adult Drug Misusers: update 2006.* London: National Treatment Agency for Substance Misuse; 2006.

29 Henry-Edwards S, Humeniuk R, Ali R, *et al.* The alcohol, smoking, and substance involvement screening test (ASSIST): guidelines for use in primary care. Draft 1.1 for Field Testing. Geneva: World Health Organization; 2003. Available at: www.who.int/substance_abuse/activities/en/Draft_The_ASSIST_Guidelines.pdf (accessed 17 February 2010).

30 Osher FC, Kofoed LL. Treatment of patients with psychiatric and psychoactive substance abuse disorders. *Hosp Community Psychiatry.* 1989; **4**: 1025–30.

31 Words of Wisdom by Buddhist philosopher Daisaku Ikeda. Available at: www.ikedaquotes.org/self-mastery.html (accessed 17 February 2010).

TO LEARN MORE

Dual Diagnosis Australia and New Zealand. Available at: www.dualdiagnosis.org.au/home

Hughes L. *Closing the Gap: a capability framework for working effectively with people with combined mental health and substance use problems*. Lincoln: Centre for Clinical and Academic Professional Innovation; 2006. Available at: www.lincoln.ac.uk/ccawi/publications/Closing%20the%20Gap.pdf

National Consortium of Consultant Nurses in Dual Diagnosis and Substance Use. Available at: www.dualdiagnosis.co.uk

CHAPTER 12

Ethics: mental health–substance use

Cynthia MA Geppert

PRE-READING EXERCISE 12.1

Time: 20 minutes

Balancing the protection of confidentiality with the need to protect the individual from harm is one of the most common conflicts encountered in the treatment of the individual with both mental health and substance use concerns and dilemmas. Often these concerns and dilemmas involve family members who are frequently placed in difficult situations, such as that illustrated in the case scenario.

Read the *case scenario,* identify the ethical issues involved and present some possible approaches to the dilemma. Consider the clinical, psychological and moral aspects of the case for the individual, his wife and you as the professional.

Case scenario

Bill is a 56-year-old auto mechanic who has been treated for major depression and alcohol dependence in a community-based integrated treatment programme. Bill has been sober for one year and is also attending a 12-step programme at his church. His depression has remitted with 100 mg of sertraline.

Recently, his supervisor indicated that there might be layoffs at the auto manufacturing plant where Bill has worked for decades. His wife Peggy now calls the clinic and tells the nurse-therapist who works with Bill that over the weekend he began drinking heavily and talking about suicide. Peggy asks that you not tell Bill she called because she is afraid he will be angry with her and perhaps become verbally abusive.

Comment

Confidentiality is an important value, but it is important for Sue to counsel Peggy during the conversation that she will likely need to disclose to Bill that Peggy is the source of her information for her to keep Bill safe. Conversely, family-centred care also means that Sue and the treatment team make every effort to also protect Peggy and to mediate a discussion between the couple.

ETHICS

This chapter will begin with a review of the major principles, virtues and concepts used to frame ethics questions and to discuss ethical issues important in clinical ethics. While these principles and virtues are significant for all healthcare their relative specification and prioritisation depends on the clinical considerations, values and wishes of the individual and other important stakeholders, and the overall contextual features of the concrete case. These unique and varied aspects of treatment especially in the complex area of mental illness–substance use may frequently generate ethical dilemmas. Ethical dilemmas are situations in which the professional cannot simultaneously, and fully, honour one or more competing ethical principles or virtues. For instance, an addiction counsellor wants to engage the family of an individual with heroin dependence in his treatment programme but the individual refuses to allow any communication. A deliberate method of working through these dilemmas can be helpful to the professional and the chapter concludes with an application of one proven means of approaching the analysis and resolution of ethical conflicts.

Ethical principles

Principles are general norms or rules that help guide ethical decision making. Beauchamp and Childress, two leaders of the school of principle-based ethics, have called them 'action guides' that help the professional identify the range of acceptable approaches in a given clinical situation.[1] *See* Table 12.1 for definitions of ethical principles and case examples.

TABLE 12.1 Important ethical principles

Principle	Definition	Case example
Autonomy	Literally 'self-rule' right of the individual to self-determination in medical decision making.	A 25-year-old college student presents to the university clinic requesting help for binge drinking which is negatively affecting his school performance.
Beneficence	To seek the good or benefit of the individual and to act to promote their well-being and interests above all other priorities.	A social worker in a substance use programme works with an individual's employer to ensure he obtains inpatient treatment for dependence on prescription pain medications without losing his job.
Confidentiality	The obligation of the professional to only release protected health information with consent of the individual or as required by law. Privacy is the right of the individual to not have his/her body or mind intruded upon without his/her consent.	A 77-year-old widower with alcohol dependence and depression calls his psychiatrist and says he is planning to kill himself. The psychiatrist calls the local authorities to bring the individual immediately to the emergency room.
Justice	Aristotle defined justice as 'to treat equals equally and unequals unequally'. In healthcare justice refers to the fair allocation of healthcare resources.	A public methadone clinic provides the medication and counselling free or on a sliding scale to people with mental health problems without income or employment.

(continued)

Principle	Definition	Case example
Nonmaleficence	The foundational duty of professionals: *primum non nocere* ['above or first of all do no harm'].	A 35-year-old veteran of the war in Afghanistan with post-traumatic stress disorder and alcohol dependence requests alprazolam to relieve his symptoms. The primary care physician instead arranges for the individual to be enrolled in a comprehensive post-traumatic stress disorder programme.
Respect for persons	Unqualified respect for the intrinsic dignity, individuality and values of a human being regardless of ethnicity, religion, sexual economic or social status or diagnosis.	A 35-year-old prostitute who has schizophrenia and cocaine dependence and is also HIV positive is welcomed with empathy and acceptance when she presents to a community mental health clinic for assistance.
Truth-telling	The prescriptive obligation to accurately and honestly disclose health information to the individual or authorised surrogates. Also the proscription not to withhold relevant facts, mislead or deceive the individual or relevant third parties.	A psychologist is treating a 35-year-old businessman for bipolar disorder and cocaine abuse. The man is on probation for shoplifting while manic and intoxicated. The individual's probation officer demands detailed therapy notes. The psychologist instead provides documentation that the individual is attending sessions and making progress.

Virtues in mental health–substance use ethics

Ethical principles provide the rational framework for thinking through complex ethical problems. Ethical virtues are qualities of character or habits of behaviour that help a person do the good, even when it is difficult, and may have adverse consequences for their own career. Principles help the head know what is right, but without virtues the heart and 'will' may find it challenging to do what is good. For instance, the disposition towards the virtues of *veracity*, which is a predisposition to tell the truth, and *compassion*, a habit of feeling another's suffering, empowers the professional to empathically but honestly tell the individual enrolled in a buprenorphine programme that his toxicology screen shows he has illicit opioids in his urine. *Fidelity* or the virtue of faithfulness enables the professional to respond to the relapse with more intensive treatment rather than discharge from care.

SELF-ASSESSMENT EXERCISE 12.1

Time: 30 minutes

An important but often neglected aspect of maintaining a high standard of professionalism is reflection on one's own moral values; how they were acquired and how they might influence practice.
- Identify the sources of your ethical values and moral virtues such as school, religion or family.

- Describe briefly what it means to you to say someone is an 'ethical person' or a 'good professional'.
- Critically assess whether you think your values and virtues are positive forces in your work with the individual or whether there may be areas where they limit or bias you.

MENTAL HEALTH–SUBSTANCE USE ETHICS

There are, however, some aspects of mental health–substance use problems and treatment that generate unique ethical conflicts, like those of stigma, or intensify dilemmas encountered in other areas of healthcare, such as confidentiality concerns.

Stigma

Stigma is *'the use of negative labels to identify a person living with mental illness'*.[2] To stigmatise individuals on the basis of a mental illness or substance use problems violates the fundamental ethical principle of respect for persons. Stigma discourages the individual from obtaining care because of fear of rejection. Discrimination negatively affects the well-being of the individual, the family and the professional.[3] Historically, mental health and substance use problems have been far more stigmatised than other medical conditions.[4] Some factors in stigmatisation are the following.

➤ Social judgements that addiction, depression and other mental illness may be at least in part voluntary and thus the individual is weak or culpable.

➤ A misunderstood and sensationalised association of mental illness and substance use with violence.

➤ In many countries drugs of use are illegal and criminalised.

➤ In some cultures the use of substances or mental illness is considered immoral.

➤ Some religious groups view both mental illness and substance use as sinful.

➤ Many persons with mental illness or substance use also have other stigmatised medical or social conditions, such as HIV and other sexually transmitted diseases, hepatitis, homelessness, or are involved in drug-dealing and prostitution, domestic violence and child abuse, suicide and homicide.

➤ Mental illness and substance use concerns and dilemmas constitute a huge social and economic burden due to unemployment, high healthcare utilisation and poverty.

➤ Many professionals receive little education about, or training in, the care of persons with mental health–substance use concerns and dilemmas, and may feel frustrated and helpless to change the chronic, relapsing and chaotic course of the disorders.

➤ The bizarre manifestations of serious mental illness and severe substance use may frighten and alienate the professional who may project their fear and disgust onto the individual.

SELF-ASSESSMENT EXERCISE 12.2

Time: 20 minutes
Review the sources of stigma for the individual with mental health–substance use concerns and dilemmas, then:

- examine your own personal views for any possible stigmatising attitudes
- analyse the treatment philosophy and routine operations of your clinical setting for both explicit and implicit expressions of stigma
- consider how can you promote a respectful, welcoming, accepting approach in all interpersonal interactions.

Confidentiality

The potential for discrimination is the primary reason mental health and even more substance use problems records in many jurisdictions and systems have higher levels of confidentiality protections than other types of medical information.[5] Professionals will frequently encounter requests from medical providers, criminal justice and public health authorities, family members, employers and insurers for information regarding the individual's treatment that may potentially undermine the therapeutic relationship and trust.[6] The following rules of thumb may be helpful in responding to such requests.

➤ Inform the individual early in all forms of care including individual and group therapy of the limitations on confidentiality.

➤ Release only the type and amount of information necessary to sufficiently respond to the request; for instance, provide only medical information not necessary in a medical emergency.

➤ When the law or the prevention of harm, such as in child abuse, requires reporting, encourage and facilitate the individual to take the lead in disclosure.

➤ Utilise closer monitoring, such as hospitalisation for a suicidal individual with substance use if this can minimise need for confidentiality breaches that could be detrimental.

SELF-ASSESSMENT EXERCISE 12.3

Time: 20 minutes

Reflect on an incident in which you feel you failed to fully protect an individual's confidentiality or you observed another professional do so.

- Distinguish between what was purposeful and what was due to thoughtlessness.
- Were there any negative consequences to this breach of confidentiality for you, the individual or your organisation?
- How could such incidents be avoided in the future?

LAW AND ETHICS

Questions of confidentiality highlight the function of the law in mental health and substance use ethics. Much more than in other areas of medical care, professionals will frequently find that legal considerations impact clinical-ethics decisions. Specific areas of interface include:

➤ involuntary commitment for mental health–substance use treatment for danger to self, other or grave passive neglect

➤ treatment refusal

➤ the role of coercion in mandating treatment

➤ treatment guardians, surrogates and conservators
➤ criminal justice involvement, such as adjudication, parole, probation, mental health courts
➤ workplace drug testing
➤ legal obligation to report child and incompetent elder abuse
➤ need to violate confidentiality to intervene in threats of suicide or homicide (Tarasoff protections).[7]

> **KEY POINT 12.1**
>
> Each jurisdiction and locality from nation to city has its own statutes, ordinances, regulations and policies. It is crucial that the professional is up to date on the relevant laws in their practice area.

When viewed from the clinical and ethical perspective, not all laws may be fair or just. Most codes of professional ethics advise the professional to respect the law while working through appropriate avenues to change legislation that does not promote the welfare of individuals.[8] For instance, many professionals, especially in Europe, would consider the attitudes of some American government officials towards harm reduction as reflecting a punitive rather than a medical response to the treatment of addiction.[9]

> **KEY POINT 12.2**
>
> Professionals should have ready access to expert legal counsel and consult them before taking any action that may be a violation of existing law.

INVOLUNTARY INTERVENTIONS AND COERCION

The ethically and clinically appropriate role and scope of mandatory or involuntary treatment, such as commitment and conservatorship for people with mental health–substance use problems, is much debated.[10] Most stakeholders, including many individuals, family and consumer advocacy groups, agree that involuntary interventions are justified and necessary when an individual with a mental illness or substance use concerns and dilemmas poses a foreseeable, realistic and serious threat of harm to self or others.[11] Within this rather black-and-white determination there are numerous grey areas where proponents argue that for severely ill people coercion can improve motivation and outcomes, and thus do good for the individual.[12] The counter-arguments of opponents of involuntary interventions claim that they may undermine the very autonomy and sense of personal responsibility that are vital to successful mental health treatment, further stigmatise the individual and threaten to undermine the therapeutic alliance.[13]

Least restrictive alternative

A useful ethico-legal concept to help balance these competing claims is that of the *least restrictive alternative*, which holds that involuntary interventions should only be utilised when all reasonable and available voluntary methods have been exhausted.[14] The proposed intervention must also have a reasonable likelihood of bringing about the desired result. An example is the use of a 'payee' for a person experiencing chronic paranoid schizophrenia who is spending the bulk of his/her disability cheque on cocaine rather than rent and food. It is realistic to believe that a payee may help the individual have sufficient monies to take care of his/her basic needs. However, for true ethical justification the payee would be one part of a comprehensive treatment plan. Whenever involuntary interventions are required they must be carried out with the utmost respect for the rights and dignity of the individual. Research suggests that this can both improve the outcome and minimise the damage to the individual.[15]

Close monitoring or intensive supervision is considered by many experts in the mental health–substance use field to be a fundamental assumption of treatment.[16] Several emerging strategies offer professionals and individuals promising alternatives to the use of traditional restrictive methods, although consensus does not exist on the more controversial measures, such as outpatient commitment. Professionals are encouraged to educate themselves regarding the ethical arguments for and against each practice:

➤ psychiatric advance directives[13]
➤ contingency management[17]
➤ outpatient commitment[18]
➤ mental health courts.[19]

KEY POINT 12.3

Professionals are encouraged to educate themselves regarding the ethical arguments for and against each practice.

DECISIONAL CAPACITY AND VOLUNTARISM

At the heart of much of the debate surrounding the place of involuntary interventions are questions of decisional capacity (*see also* Book 2, Chapter 15). *See* Box 12.1 for the elements of decisional capacity.[20]

BOX 12.1 Elements of decisional capacity

1 The capacity to clearly communicate a choice.
2 The capacity to comprehend information such as risks, benefits and alternatives of a proposed treatment.
3 The capacity to reason about facts to arrive at a logical and consistent conclusion.
4 The capacity to appreciate and make authentic choices that meaningfully reflect one's values.

Decisional capacity traditionally has had a cognitive emphasis but for the individual with mental illness and substance use problems, the volitional and appreciative components of decision making may be even more vital and potentially diminished by their conditions. Voluntarism refers to the free and full participation of an individual in treatment decisions and implies the absence of significant internal and external coercion. *See* Table 12.2 for Robert's four domains with case examples.[21,22]

TABLE 12.2 Domains of voluntarism[21,22]

Domain	Example
Developmental factors	A 78-year-old with mild dementia, generalised anxiety disorder and benzodiazepine misuse has impairments in working memory that interfere with his ability to manage his medications and participate in cognitive behavioural therapy.
Illness-related considerations	A 75-year-old grandmother with major depression and over-use of prescription opioids may be so depressed that she refuses further treatment, thinking it is hopeless.
Psychological issues and cultural and religious factors	His church counsellor tells a 32-year-old individual with schizophrenia and alcohol dependence that he should not take psychiatric medications because they are a 'crutch'.
External features and pressures	The husband of a 45-year-old mother of three who has been diagnosed with bipolar disorder and cocaine dependence tells his wife that if she does not enter an inpatient rehabilitation programme he will divorce her and seek custody of their children.

Decisional capacity and voluntarism are necessary for informed consent for treatment and research and preconditions for legal and moral responsibility. Research has shown that some individuals with serious mental illnesses, such as schizophrenia and early dementia, may have clinically significant impairments in decisional capacity.[23,24] Increasingly, studies are also finding cognitive deficiencies in individuals with substance use problems that may adversely affect their ability to make decisions in their own best interests.[25] If professionals, families have concerns about an individual's decisional capacity or voluntarism they have an ethical obligation to perform request an appropriate assessment.[22,26] A number of validated instruments are available and professionals should seek expert neuropsychiatric consultation if indicated.[27]

> **KEY POINT 12.4**

Decisional capacity is task specific: individuals may be able to make some medical treatment decisions but not financial ones.

Professionals have a duty to try to ameliorate deficits or enhance strengths whenever possible through a variety of options:
➤ use of educational enhancements such as audiovisual and computerised aids[28,29]
➤ brief cognitive interventions to improve understanding[30]
➤ repeating information and providing several trials for comprehension[31]
➤ adjustment of medications to better control symptoms
➤ substance use treatment

➤ use of surrogate decision makers when decisional capacity cannot be sufficiently addressed.[32]

A MODEL FOR DECISION MAKING

Reading this chapter may make you feel somewhat uncertain, or even overwhelmed, at the prospect of decision making regarding the complex, nuanced and challenging ethical dilemmas presented. As with clinical decision making, having a structured and systematic method, such as the 'Four Box' method, can help us arrive at a sound and balanced judgement.[33] *See* Table 12.3 for adaptation of the model and associated ethical principles.

TABLE 12.3 Decision-making model

Topic	Principles
Medical indications • Mental health and substance use diagnosis, prognosis • Chronic, acute or crisis situation? • Goals of treatment, likelihood of success and back-up plans.	• Nonmaleficence: minimising harm to the individual • Beneficence: maximising individual benefit.
Individual preferences • Decisional capacity • Treatment preferences • Adequacy of informed consent process • Surrogate decision maker needed or available • Advance directives • Is the individual refusing or unable to participate in treatment?	• Autonomy • Respect for persons.
Interests of other parties / contextual features • Are there family issues that are important to or may influence decisions? • Are there team concerns or dynamics that may impact treatment decisions? • What is the bearing of the law on the case? • Are confidentiality limits or concerns present? • Are there economic or financial factors involved or possible conflicts of interest? • Are religious and/or cultural factors important contextual features? • Are resource allocation problems limiting treatment options? • Is there potential professional or system stigmatisation of the individual?	• Justice • Fiduciary relationship • Fidelity • Confidentiality • Veracity.

POST-READING EXERCISE 12.1

Time: 30 minutes
Use the decision-making model at the end of the chapter to work through a clinical-ethics dilemma you recently encountered in your practice.

REFERENCES

1 Beauchamp TL, Childress JF. *Principles of Biomedical Ethics*. 6th ed. New York, NY: Oxford University Press; 2009.
2 Substance Abuse and Mental Health Services Administration. *Anti-Stigma: do you know the facts*. Rockville, MD; 2003 (cited 18 July 2009). Available at: http://mentalhealth.samhsa.gov/publications/allpubs/OEL99–0004/default.asp (accessed 18 February 2010).
3 Link BG, Struening EL, Rahav M, *et al*. On stigma and its consequences: evidence from a longitudinal study of men with dual diagnoses of mental illness and substance abuse. *J Health Soc Behav*. 1997; **38**: 177–90.
4 Bogenschutz MP. Caring for persons with addictions. In: Roberts LW, Dyer AR, editors. *Concise Guide to Ethics in Mental Health Care*. Washington, DC: American Psychiatric Publishing; 2004.
5 Brooks MK. Legal aspects of confidentiality and individual information. In: Lowinson JH, Ruiz P, Millman RB, *et al*., editors. *Substance Abuse: a comprehensive textbook*. 4th ed. Philadelphia, PA: Lippincott Williams & Wilkins; 2005. pp. 1361–82.
6 Roberts LW, Geppert C, Bailey R. Ethics in psychiatric practice: informed consent, the therapeutic relationship, and confidentiality. *J Psychiatr Pract*. 2002; **8**: 290–305.
7 Gavaghan C. A Tarasoff for Europe? A European human rights perspective on the duty to protect. *Int J Law Psychiatry*. 2007; **30**: 255–67.
8 American Medical Association Council on Ethical and Judicial Affairs. *Code of Medical Ethics: current opinions with annotations*. Chicago, IL: American Medical Association; 2006–7.
9 Tammi T, Hurme T. How the harm reduction movement contrasts itself against punitive prohibition. *Int J Drug Policy*. 2007; **18**: 84–7.
10 Sullivan MA, Birkmayer F, Boyarsky BK, *et al*. Uses of coercion in addiction treatment: clinical aspects. *Am J Addict*. 2008; **17**: 36–47.
11 National Alliance on Mental Illness Board of Directors. *Policy on Involuntary Committment and Court-Ordered Treatment*. Arlington, VA: National Alliance on Mental Illness; 1995.
12 Nace EP, Birkmayer F, Sullivan MA, *et al*. Socially sanctioned coercion mechanisms for addiction treatment. *Am J Addict*. 2007; **16**: 15–23.
13 Swanson JW, Tepper MC, Backlar P, *et al*. Psychiatric advance directives: an alternative to coercive treatment? *Psychiatry*. 2000; **63**: 160–72.
14 Appelbaum PS, Gutheil TG. *Clinical Handbook of Psychiatry and the Law*. 2nd ed. Philadelphia, PA: Lippincott, Williams & Wilkins; 2007.
15 Noordsy DL, Mercer CC, Drake RE. Involuntary interventions in dual disorders programs. In: Backlar P, Cutler D, editors. *Ethics in Community Mental Health Care*. New York, NY: Kluwer; 2002. pp. 95–115.
16 Center for Substance Abuse Treatment. Substance abuse treatment for persons with co-ocurring disorders. In: *Administration SAMHS*. Rockville, MD: Center for Substance Abuse Treatment; 2005.
17 Kirby KC, Benishek LA, Dugosh KL, *et al*. Substance abuse treatment providers' beliefs and objections regarding contingency management: implications for dissemination. *Drug Alcohol Depend*. 2006; **85**: 19–27.
18 Munetz MR, Galon PA, Frese FJ, III. The ethics of mandatory community treatment. *J Am Acad Psychiatry Law*. 2003; **31**: 173–83.
19 Schneider RD. Mental health courts. *Curr Opin Psychiatry*. 2008; **21**: 510–3.
20 Appelbaum PS. Clinical practice. Assessment of individuals' competence to consent to treatment. *N Engl J Med*. 2007; **357**: 1834–40.
21 Roberts LW. Informed consent and the capacity for voluntarism. *Am J Psychiatry*. 2002; **159**: 705–12.

22 Geppert CM, Abbott C. Voluntarism in consultation psychiatry: the forgotten capacity. *Am J Psychiatry*. 2007; **164**: 409–13.

23 Palmer BW, Dunn LB, Appelbaum PS, *et al*. Correlates of treatment-related decision-making capacity among middle-aged and older individuals with schizophrenia. *Arch Gen Psychiatry*. 2004; **61**: 230–6.

24 Gurrera RJ, Moye J, Karel MJ, *et al*. Cognitive performance predicts treatment decisional abilities in mild to moderate dementia. *Neurology*. 2006; **66**: 1367–72.

25 Kalivas PW, Volkow ND. The neural basis of addiction: a pathology of motivation and choice. *Am J Psychiatry*. 2005; **162**: 1403–13.

26 Jeste DV, Saks E. Decisional capacity in mental illness and substance use disorders: empirical database and policy implications. *Behav Sci Law*. 2006; **24**: 607–28.

27 Dunn LB, Nowrangi MA, Palmer BW, *et al*. Assessing decisional capacity for clinical research or treatment: a review of instruments. *Am J Psychiatry*. 2006; **163**: 1323–34.

28 Jeste DV, Dunn LB, Folsom DP, *et al*. Multimedia educational aids for improving consumer knowledge about illness management and treatment decisions: a review of randomized controlled trials. *J Psychiatr Res*. 2008; **42**: 1–21.

29 Dunn LB, Lindamer LA, Palmer BW, *et al*. Enhancing comprehension of consent for research in older individuals with psychosis: a randomized study of a novel consent procedure. *Am J Psychiatry*. 2001; **158**: 1911–13.

30 Moser DJ, Reese RL, Hey CT, *et al*. Using a brief intervention to improve decisional capacity in schizophrenia research. *Schizophr Bull*. 2006; **32**: 116–20.

31 Wirshing DA, Wirshing WC, Marder SR, *et al*. Informed consent: assessment of comprehension. *Am J Psychiatry*. 1998; **155**: 1508–11.

32 High DM. Surrogate decision making. Who will make decisions for me when I can't? *Clin Geriatr Med*. 1994; **10**: 445–62.

33 Jonsen AR, Seigler M, Winslade WJ. *Clinical Ethics: a practical approach to ethical decisions in clinical medicine*. 6th ed. New York, NY: McGraw-Hill; 2006.

TO LEARN MORE

Backlar P, Cutler DL, editors. *Ethics in Community Mental Health Care*. New York, NY: Kluwer; 2002.

Centre for Addiction and Mental Health (CAMH), Bioethics Service. Available at: www.jointcentre forbioethics.ca/partners/camh.shtml

Geppert CMA, Roberts LW. *The Book of Ethics Expert Guidance for Professionals Who Treat Addiction*. Center City, MN: Hazelden; 2008.

Roberts LW, Dyer AR, editors. *Ethics in Mental Health Care*. Washington, DC: American Psychiatric Press; 2004.

Roberts LW, Hoop JG, editors. *Professionalism and Ethics: Q & A Self-study Guide for Mental Health Professionals*. Washington, DC: American Psychiatric Press; 2008.

CHAPTER 13

Brain injury, mental health–substance use

Chris Holmwood

INTRODUCTION

Acquired brain injury, substance use and mental health problems frequently occur together. People with this mix of problems present clinicians, health and social service managers and at times the criminal justice system with a range of challenges. All three types of condition, acquired brain injury, mental disorder and substance use problems, affect emotions, cognitions and behaviour. The management of the different health concerns is highly interdependent.

The link between structural brain damage, personality and behaviour only emerged as a possibility in the mid 1800s. Among the triggers for this was a report concerning a Phineas Gage.[1] Mr Gage, was a railway worker. In an accident due to a premature detonation of blasting powder, a 30 mm diameter metal tamping rod was driven through his right frontal lobe. After surviving the initial injury, itself a subject of much interest at the time, he then experienced significant and permanent personality change. This report began to stimulate a deeper appreciation of the structure of the brain, in particular with respect to personality and behaviour.

Brain injury can occur as a result of trauma, toxic insult, hypoxia, and metabolite deficiencies, such as hypoglycaemia and thiamine deficiency. Traumatic brain injury is more common in people with substance use problems and in those with mental health–substance use problems. Substances themselves can cause brain injury either directly (e.g. alcohol, volatile solvents), or indirectly (e.g. stroke secondary to hypertension from alcohol, cocaine or methamphetamine use). Hypoxia or hypoglycaemia related to overdose of alcohol, benzodiazepines, opioids or other sedatives will result in brain injury. Such injury is sometimes termed substance-related brain injury. Chronic high alcohol intake is often associated with thiamine deficiency, which itself compounds direct alcohol-related toxicity. Alcohol-related brain injury is probably the most common substance-related brain injury (a subset of acquired brain injury; *see* Figure 13.1).

Many people presenting with substance use problems will have cognitive impairment from a range of causes. The causes are multi-factorial and the severity will vary. The key is to determine what the person's disability is, and try to implement strategies that will reduce that disability, improve their quality of life while helping to maintain as much independence as possible.

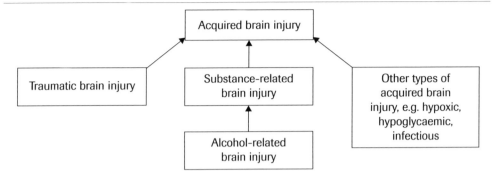

FIGURE 13:1 Types of acquired brain injury

SELF-ASSESSMENT EXERCISE 13.1

Time: 10 minutes
- As a professional, how would you determine a person's quality of life?
- What formal scales are you aware of to determine a person's quality of life?
- What are the advantages of these scales?
- Where, on a scale of 0–10, would you rate your quality of life (0=worst 10=best)

There are several questions around prevalence, detection and diagnosis, and providing care for people with mental health–substance use problems that need to be answered before there can be an effective response on a health and social service level.

Q: DOES SUBSTANCE USE PREDISPOSE TO BRAIN INJURY (OTHER THAN SUBSTANCE-RELATED BRAIN INJURY)?

 TIME OUT: Take five minutes to reflect on this question. Make notes of your conclusions before reading on.

Traumatic brain injury is common among people with substance use problems. Antecedent substance use problems are common among people with traumatic brain injury.

Case study: Part 1
Malcolm, age 42, married man
Malcolm has a 25-year history of heavy drinking and depression. He has worked all his adult life in the insurance industry. He has never drunk at work but after work drinks 3 litres of beer every night. One night when intoxicated he fell and fractured his forearm, consequently needing open reduction and internal fixation. Two days after the accident he developed alcohol withdrawal in hospital. Malcolm's withdrawal was fortunately recognised early and was managed with diazepam and thiamine, overseen by the hospital liaison alcohol and drug unit. He was discharged home on day 10.

SELF-ASSESSMENT EXERCISE 13.2

Time: 5 minutes
Considering Malcolm's case study so far, what is the probability that Malcolm has some underlying cognitive impairment?

Brain injury can result from a number of factors. Trauma is one cause. While not particularly relevant now, Malcolm could well have sustained a significant head injury from the fall, instead of a broken arm. Two in three people with substance use problems have been found to have had previous head injury.[2,3] The relationship between substance use and head injury is strong. The substance use will increase the risk of traumatic brain injury directly from accidents and from intentional self-injury. In addition, substance use and traumatic head injury may have common antecedents. For instance, underlying personality traits, such as impulsivity and novelty seeking, may increase the risk of both trauma and substance use.

While the relationship between alcohol use and cognitive impairment across the population is complex, there is no doubt that at high alcohol intake levels, direct alcohol-related brain injury is related to the cumulative dose. In addition, thiamine deficiency augments the risk, so people with poor diets who drink heavily are at increased risk.[4] Malcolm is at risk of acquired brain injury purely because of his alcohol use (due to increased risk of trauma and direct effect of the alcohol). Conversely, Malcolm has been supported by his wife and his diet has been quite balanced (apart from the 3 litres of beer per day) over the years, so his risk of thiamine deficiency associated Wernicke–Korsakoff syndrome is reduced.

Q: DO MENTAL HEALTH PROBLEMS PREDISPOSE TO ACQUIRED BRAIN INJURY?

 TIME OUT: Take five minutes to reflect on this question. Make notes of your conclusions before reading on.

Primary mental disorders can lead to suicide or self-harm attempts that can result in brain injury.[5] Uncompleted hangings, drug overdoses, intentional motor vehicle crashes and other high lethality suicidal actions can result in traumatic, toxic or hypoxic brain injury.[6] Substance use problems are closely linked with suicidal behaviours, regardless of the presence of a primary mental illness, resulting in the same risk of acquired brain injury.[7]

KEY POINT 13.1

Certain personality traits or problems (in particular some of the Diagnostic and Statistical Manual of Mental Disorders [DSM] 4, cluster B, personality problems) characterised by impulsivity, recklessness and emotional volatility lead to risky behaviour that may result in brain injury[8] – as well as substance use.

Q: DOES BRAIN INJURY PRECIPITATE OR EXACERBATE SUBSTANCE USE PROBLEMS?

 TIME OUT: Take five minutes to reflect on this question. Make notes of your conclusions before reading on.

There is a mixed picture here with some holding that rates of substance use actually decline after a brain injury is sustained, and some that it increases.

There seem to be some time-related patterns with people using substances more in the period after the injury but reducing after that.[3,9] Lack of access to substances – due to the physical disability from the brain injury – may also confound the findings in those people with more severe brain injury. Conversely, those with less severe brain injury may be able to access alcohol and other substances more easily post-injury, reverting to problematic use.

In addition, people with acquired brain injury may be more sensitive to substances. Therefore, levels of use that might be considered low risk in people without a brain injury may present a higher risk.

> **Case study: Part 2**
> Malcolm returns to drinking his beer each night. Six months later he has another fall in the bathroom one night and sustains a closed head injury. He is unconscious for 20 minutes. CT scan shows some diffuse oedema of the left frontal and temporal lobes. While under observation he goes into withdrawal again. He is managed as an inpatient, spending 10 days in hospital. By the time he leaves hospital he seems to have had about 12 hours of post-traumatic amnesia. Malcolm has some problems with remembering names and events but after three weeks in rehabilitation (and abstinence), he is able to go home and resume work.

Q: DOES BRAIN INJURY PRECIPITATE OR EXACERBATE MENTAL HEALTH PROBLEMS?

 TIME OUT: Take five minutes to reflect on this question. Make notes of your conclusions before reading on.

Brain injury results in a lifetime increase in suicide risk,[8,10] and the professional needs to consider this with every encounter. Depression is common and may emerge at any stage post-injury. Anxiety problems (especially post-traumatic stress disorder, panic disorder) can emerge as a result of the injury event itself, or obsessive–compulsive disorder can develop as the person tries to adjust to cognitive deficits. The emergence of depression can adversely affect function in people with a history of head injury.[11]

Case study: Part 3

Since his return to work, Malcolm has been less energetic and less engaged in life than before his injury. He socialises less. He has been able to manage with work but his supervisor and colleagues are worried about him. Currently, Malcolm feels flat but denies any thoughts of wanting to end his life. Now, for the first time in 25 years, he has not drunk any alcohol for three months.

It is difficult to know whether Malcolm's current presentation is due to depression, due to the cognitive effect of the traumatic brain injury, or a direct cumulative effect of alcohol on the brain, or all three.

Q: WHAT IS THE BEST APPROACH TO ASSESSING PEOPLE WITH POSSIBLE BRAIN INJURY, MENTAL HEALTH PROBLEMS AND SUBSTANCE USE?

 TIME OUT: Take five minutes to reflect on this question. Make notes of your conclusions before reading on.

Prognosis after traumatic brain injury is highly variable. Predictors of poorer prognosis include longer duration of unconsciousness, longer duration of post-traumatic amnesia (both indicative of severity of injury), and lower pre-injury function. Similarly, the presence of pre-injury mental health problems and problems related to substance use-also affect the incidence of these problems post injury.

Ongoing assessment of mental state

Given that mental health problems are common after brain injury,[2] ongoing assessments should be undertaken, in order to detect emerging mental health problems that may be responsive to treatment. However, intoxication may make assessments of people with this range of problems particularly challenging.

The first step in the mental health assessment, determining the person's level of intoxication (which may be subtle or not so subtle), is important. Assessment of the intoxicated person can be difficult and may be reduced (for a time at least) to assessing risk to self and others.

In addition, there is some overlap between behavioural features of brain injury and the vegetative features of depression. Differentiate between the two by exploring the cognitions and emotions of the individual, to check for congruence. Feelings of hopelessness, worthlessness and anhedonia (an inability to experience pleasure from a normally pleasurable situation), which are more specific features of depression, should be looked for by the clinician.[12,13] In particular, monitoring of warning signs for risk of suicide is important, including:

➤ thoughts of hopelessness
➤ suicidal ideation[10]
➤ failure to adjust to life following brain injury.

Case study: Part 4
In Malcolm's case, he denies feelings of worthlessness, or hopelessness. He is not tearful. He lacks energy and isn't getting much enjoyment out of life at present. He used to enjoy the social aspects of work, the challenge of working with new clients and getting new contracts. Malcolm says that his concentration is not as good as it was. His sleep is still disturbed, with some vivid dreams every night, some of which are frightening. He does not have early morning wakening, but his sleep remains restless and unrefreshing.

Malcolm's presentation may be due to multiple factors, and it is judged that he is not depressed, but rather is still recovering from the head injury, the adjustment to being alcohol free, and possibly from the longer term effects of the alcohol.

Assessment of cognitive impairment
Assessment of cognitive impairment is often done in an opportunistic manner when the person is seen in a non-intoxicated state. Cognitive impairment at any particular time may be due to:
➤ intoxication
➤ prolonged but reversible neurological damage
➤ longer-term irreversible structural brain damage related to the substance use (e.g. Wernicke–Korsakoff syndrome), hypoxia or trauma. However, even the notion of irreversible brain injury has now come into question as it is being increasingly recognised that the brain is plastic (plasticity, or neuroplasticity, is the ability of the brain to reorganise neural pathways based on new experiences), and can compensate for deficits to a greater or lesser degree.

There are several assessment instruments that can be used to assess brain function in the clinical setting where substance use is a problem. These should be administered by a competent professional. While such assessments can help to unlock some specifics of the dysfunction, and can inform more specific types of treatments and ways of responding to more challenging behaviours, they need to be validated against an assessment of 'how' the person functions in their familiar environment. This determines the level of disability and can provide some direction as to the types of support services and aids that might be required. Directly observing the person in their own environment can be the quickest and most valid way of assessing their level of function. While time intensive, the assessment will have high face validity. The assessment needs to include observation of the:
➤ state of the person's accommodation
➤ levels of hygiene
➤ food procurement and preparation
➤ interpersonal relations
➤ ability to plan and operationalise outings, financial transactions.

SELF-ASSESSMENT EXERCISE 13.3

Time: 15 minutes
- Is there any other information you would find helpful? Consider physical, psychological, emotional, spiritual elements.
- Consider the problems that are common in people with substance use-related brain injury.

Alcohol-related brain injury represents a spectrum of disability, with some people being impaired but able to compensate and function adequately. Verbal functioning tends to be maintained, leading to premature exclusion of impairment as a possibility.

Alcohol-related brain injury can be divided into two categories:
1   Wernicke–Korsakoff syndrome where the damage is mediated through thiamine deficiency.
2   A more global brain syndrome.[15]

The longer-term features of Wernicke–Korsakoff syndrome are anterograde memory impairment and deficits in abstraction and problem solving. The features of non-Wernicke–Korsakoff-type alcohol-related cognitive impairment are slowed information processing, difficulty learning new material, difficulties with abstraction and problem solving, and visuospatial difficulties.

Common problems in people with substance use-related brain injury

➤ Goal setting, planning, organising, thinking through consequences, decision making.
➤ Reacting to environmental changes, flexibility in thinking, learning from mistakes, solving novel problems resulting in routinised or repetitive behaviour.
➤ Lack of spontaneity, blunted affect, lack of motivation but in some circumstances lack of impulse control.
➤ Poor social skills with difficulty perceiving another's view and not being able to understand how his/her behaviour affects others.
➤ Low frustration threshold and decreased ability to control anger expression. This may at times spill over into uncharacteristic aggression.
➤ Processing information, word finding.
➤ Short-term memory problems may also present, exacerbating all the above and resulting in further disorientation. Memory problems point strongly to Wernicke–Korsakoff syndrome.

Some of these features can be seen in the context of traumatic brain injury and hypoxic brain injury so establishing aetiology is not always possible. Many features can be discerned from observing the individual in his/her environment or from descriptions of problems from the individual, the family, neighbours or other professionals.

Assessment of substance use in people with brain injury can be difficult due to impaired memory. A comprehensive assessment will include a clinical face to face assessment with the person.[16] However, memory problems may make this assessment less valid. In addition, in some situations, the person will have been referred by another professional, may not want to be assessed, and, therefore, may be uncooperative.

The following can be used to validate the clinical assessment and to provide further additional information:

➤ an examination of bio-markers related to substance use
➤ information from family, friends, neighbours, other professionals, where available
➤ review of previous health and other records.

Q: WHAT IS THE BEST APPROACH TO PROVIDING CARE FOR PEOPLE WITH BRAIN INJURY, MENTAL HEALTH PROBLEMS AND SUBSTANCE USE?

 TIME OUT: Take five minutes to reflect on this question. Make notes of your conclusions before reading on.

Responding to the cognitive impairment

Cognitive improvement post brain injury can continue for up to two years post injury.[17] While some of this recovery is time dependent and occurs as a result of neurophysiological 'repair', some of the recovery is also thought to be due to experiences the person has after the injury. With contemporary views about brain plasticity, the traditional separation of brain 'structure' and 'function' is now becoming obsolete, with the two being tightly interdependent.

There would appear be a role for cognitive-based programmes, which have shown to improve some outcomes, such as levels of anxiety, self-concept, and personal relationships. However, beneficial effects on health or employment-related outcomes have not been demonstrated.[18–20] There is a spectrum of severity of cognitive impairment associated with acquired brain injury and the person's capacity to engage in cognitive interventions will vary with the level of severity.

It is generally considered that rehabilitation from the brain injury is hampered by ongoing substance use and vice versa. However, there is a range of interventions that can help to improve people's quality of life that to some degree may be independent of their ongoing substance use. Some examples are as follows.

➤ **Memory aids**: whiteboards with the day's programme or lists of tasks, wristwatch alarms, memory notebooks and programmed reminder devices.
➤ **Basic behavioural strategies**: structuring a small range of activities that are accessible, enjoyable and rewarding.
➤ **Memory training using skills**: which enhances information retention. These might include the person:
  — repeating instructions to check that they have understood the advice given
  — repeating new acquaintance's names frequently in early conversation in order to better remember the name
  — asking for the instructions or advice to be repeated to consolidate recall.
➤ **Maps**: attendance at appointments can be assisted using maps, and the memory aids mentioned above.

Many of these approaches require significant input from other people, such as family, friends, or support services. Despite the reliance of some input by others they do enable improved independence.

Addressing substance use

Most interventions for substance use involve significant cognitive skills. Ability to reflect on the effects the substance use has on the individual and others around them, recognition of the need to change, forward planning, contingency management and the execution of these plans are all areas that are affected through brain injury.

Despite these drawbacks, motivational interviewing should be utilised whenever possible, where there is ambivalence about substance use. There is some evidence that Motivational Interviewing works to reduce substance use in people with acquired brain injury and problematic substance use.[21] These effects will be more effective with non-dependent substance use. Such programmes probably need to be persistent, structured and have some degree of repetition in order to compensate for impaired cognitive abilities of the individual.

In addition, case management has been demonstrated to improve outcomes in terms of employment and community integration for this group.[22] In light of the comments above about the need for third parties (family members, friends, other support services) to be engaged, and the sometimes broad range of services needed, the role of case management in optimising coordination of care is self-evident.

Assisting with mental health problems

Suicide is a significant risk. Monitoring and responding to suicide risk is an important task for all professionals involved in the care of people with acquired brain injury, and related mental health–substance use problems. There is considerable evidence that the risk of self-harm after traumatic brain injury does not diminish with time, so the need for vigilance persists.[8,10,23] Given the additional risk of suicide associated with underlying mental problems and substance use problems, the professional needs to be vigilant.

Treatment of mental illness in people with an underlying brain injury requires a flexible approach. Teasing out the diagnostic formulation with all its overlaps and ambiguities requires some acceptance of uncertainty.

As mentioned above with respect to the management of substance use problems, depending on the level of cognitive impairment, cognitive approaches may be useful. For example, active treatment of anxiety problems following mild to moderate brain injury has been shown to be helpful.[24]

When cognitive strategies cannot be used, pharmacological agents should be considered. The risk-benefit analysis for use of medications is sometimes unclear. People with brain injury may experience side-effects more frequently, and may not tolerate these as well. In addition, clinical improvement may not be as clear-cut. The use of sertraline (a selective serotonin reuptake inhibitor) has been shown to be effective in treating depression in people with an acquired brain injury.[25,26]

The risk–benefit ratio of any interventions in this group varies considerably. In addition, rates of self-harm are relatively high. There is a need for closer monitoring of progress, with special attention paid to side-effects of treatment, and to assessment of treatment adherence.

Supportive intervention

The degree of support required for people with brain injury, and mental-substance use problems, will vary with the level of function.

There is some evidence that case management improves outcomes. If intra- and interdisciplinary professionals and family are involved, coordination of these activities needs to occur. Case management involves the following functions:

➤ assessment
➤ planning
➤ linking
➤ monitoring
➤ advocacy
➤ individual identification and outreach.[27]

SELF-ASSESSMENT EXERCISE 13.4

Time: 15 minutes
Make a list of the type of supportive intervention(s) you think would help maintaining independence. Consider the individual, family and other professionals.

Supportive intervention(s) that can help to keep people independent include help with the following.

➤ **Accommodation**: the individual may not be able to access private rental and or may have special needs.
➤ **Activities of daily living**: making appointments, shopping, food preparation, etc.
➤ **Vocational support**: engaging the individual in meaningful work-related activities that brings him/her into contact with other people will assist with self-esteem, with daily activity scheduling and (if paid work) the financial status.
➤ **Family engagement and support**: is highly valued but the reality in many situations is that the individual is alienated from the family. Family carers need to be protected. They need regular breaks built into their weekly schedules. Longer term respite needs to be available on a regular basis.
➤ **Drug-free recreational activities**: just as for work-related activities, enjoyable recreational activities, especially if regularly scheduled, can assist with quality of life. In the context of people with substance use problems, recreational environments free of alcohol or drugs are important.
➤ **Appointment of a legal guardian**: to assist with management of finances and other aspects of decision making.

CONCLUSION

Brain injury, mental disorders and substance use problems frequently occur together. There is significant overlap in their clinical presentations. People with this range of problems require careful assessment with corroboration of interview findings with biochemical markers, brain imaging at times, as well as information from families and friends, and other health and social services. Professionals must always be aware of the risk of suicide.

The complexity of brain injury, mental health–substance use problems will adversely affect the outcome of each other.

A range of specific interventions can be useful. These include:
➤ motivational interviewing
➤ programmes to assist cognitive impairment
➤ memory assisting aids
➤ activity structuring
➤ cognitive approaches for anxiety
➤ judicious use of pharmacotherapy for identified mental problems, such as depression and anxiety problems.

KEY POINT 13.2

Cognitive programmes need to be adapted to the individual impairments of the participants.

In addition, supportive intervention can assist the individual with brain injury and mental health–substance use problems maintain independence and a reasonable quality of life.

REFERENCES
1 Barker FG. Phineas among the phrenologists: the American crowbar case and nineteenth-century theories of cerebral localization. *J Neurosurg.* 1995; **82**: 672–82.
2 Deb S, Lyons I, Koutzoukis C, *et al.* Rate of psychiatric illness 1 year after traumatic brain injury. *Am J Psychiatry.* 1999; **156**: 374–8.
3 Hibbard MR, Uysal S, Kepler K, *et al.* Axis I psychopathology in individuals with traumatic brain injury. *J Head Trauma Rehabil.* 1998; **13**: 24–39.
4 Berman M. Severe brain dysfunction: alcoholic Korsakoff's syndrome. *Alcohol Health Res World.* 1990; **14**: 120–9.
5 Mann JJ, Waternaux C, Haas GL, *et al.* Toward a clinical model of suicidal behavior in psychiatric patients. *Am J Psychiatry.* 1999; **156**: 181–9.
6 Fann JR, Leonetti A, Jaffe K, *et al.* Psychiatric illness and subsequent traumatic brain injury: a case control study. *J Neurol Neurosurg Psychiatry.* 2002; **72**: 615–20.
7 Johnston A, Pirkis J, Burgess P. Suicidal thoughts and behaviors among Australian adults: findings from the 2007 National Survey of Mental Health and Wellbeing. *Aust N Z J Psychiatry.* 2009; **43**: 635–43.
8 Teasdale TW, Engberg AW. Suicide after traumatic brain injury: a population study. *J Neurol Neurosurg Psychiatry.* 2001; **71**: 436–40.
9 Koponen S, Taiminen T, Portin R, *et al.* Axis I and II psychiatric problems after traumatic brain injury: a 30-year follow-up study. *Am J Psychiatry.* 2002; **159**: 1315–21.
10 Simpson G, Tate R. Suicidality after traumatic brain injury: demographic, injury and clinical correlates. *Psychol Med.* 2002; **32**: 687–97.
11 Hibbard MR, Ashman TA, Spielman LA, *et al.* Relationship between depression and psychosocial functioning after traumatic brain injury. *Arch Phys Med Rehabil.* 2004; **85**: S43–S53.
12 Simpson GK, Tate RL. Preventing suicide after traumatic brain injury: implications for general practice. *Med J Aust.* 2007; **187**: 229–32.

13 Seel RT, Kreutzer JS, Rosenthal M, *et al*. Depression after traumatic brain injury: a National Institute on Disability and Rehabilitation Research Model Systems multicenter investigation. *Arch Phys Med Rehabil.* 2003; **84**: 177–84.

14 Goldman M. Recovery of cognitive function in alcoholics: the relationship to treatment. *Alcohol Health Res World.* 1995; **19**: 148–54.

15 Evert DL, Oscar-Berman M. Alcohol-related cognitive impairments: an overview of how alcoholism may affect the workings of the brain. *Alcohol Health Res World.* 1995; **19**: 89–96.

16 Taylor LA, Kreutzner JS, Demm SR, *et al*. Traumatic brain injury and substance abuse: a review and analysis of the literature. *Neuropsychol Rehabil.* 2003; **13**: 165–88.

17 Schretlen DJ, Shapiro AM. A quantitative review of the effects of traumatic brain injury on cognitive functioning. *Int Rev Psychiatry.* 2003; **15**: 341–9.

18 Carney N, Chesnut RM, Maynard H, *et al*. Effect of cognitive rehabilitation on outcomes for persons with traumatic brain injury: a systematic review. *J Head Trauma Rehabil.* 1999; **14**: 277–307.

19 Chesnut RM, Carney N, Maynard H, *et al*. Rehabilitation for traumatic brain injury. Evidence Report/Technology Assessment 2. Rockville, MD: Agency for Health Care Policy and Research; 1998. Available at: www.ncbi.nlm.nih.gov/books/bv.fcgi?rid=hstat1.chapter.84262 (accessed 19 February 2010).

20 Cicerone KD, Dahlberg C, Kalmar K, *et al*. Evidence-based cognitive rehabilitation: recommendations for clinical practice. *Arch Phys Med Rehabil.* 2000; **81**: 1596–615.

21 Cox WM, Heinemann AW, Miranti SV, *et al*. Outcomes of systematic motivational counselling for substance use following traumatic brain injury. *J Addict Dis.* 2003; **22**: 93–110.

22 Heinemann AW, Corrigan JD, Moore D. Case management for traumatic brain injury survivors with alcohol problems. *Rehabil Psychol.* 2004; **49**: 156–66.

23 Anstey KJ, Butterworth P, Jorm AF, *et al*. A population survey found an association between self-reports of traumatic brain injury and increased psychiatric symptoms. *J Clin Epidemiol.* 2004; **57**: 1202–9.

24 Soo C, Tate R. Psychological treatment for anxiety in people with traumatic brain injury. *Cochrane Database Syst Rev.* 2007; CD005239.

25 Lee H, Kim SW, Kim JM, *et al*. Comparing effects of methylphenidate, sertraline and placebo on neuropsychiatric sequelae in patients with traumatic brain injury. *Hum Psychopharmacol.* 2005; **20**: 97–104.

26 Fann JR, Uomoto JM, Katon WJ. Sertraline in the treatment of major depression following mild traumatic brain injury. *J Neuropsychiatry Clin Neurosci.* 2000; **12**: 226–32.

27 Graham K, Timney CB. Case management in addictions treatment. *J Subst Abuse Treat.* 1990; **7**: 181–6.

TO LEARN MORE

Gordon A. *Comorbidity of Mental Problems and Substance Use: a brief guide for the primary care clinician.* Barton, ACT: Department of Health and Ageing; 2009. Available at: www.nationaldrugstrategy.gov.au/internet/drugstrategy/publishing.nsf/Content/mono71

Trevena L, Cameron I, Porwal M. *Clinical Practice Guidelines for the Care of People Living with Traumatic Brain Injury in the Community.* Full Report. Sydney, NSW: University of Sydney; 2004. Available at: www.health.usyd.edu.au/shdg/docs/Clinical_Prac_Guidelines_TBI_Full_report.pdf

ACKNOWLEDGEMENT
The author of this chapter would like to thank Mr Rin Minniti, Senior Clinical Psychologist, at Drug and Alcohol Services South Australia for his advice on this manuscript

CHAPTER 14

Heatwave, mental health–substance use

Lynette Cusack, Charlotte de Crespigny and Peter Athanasos

PRE-READING EXERCISE 14.1

Time: 10 minutes

Consider the implications of heatwave and mental health–substance use. List what problems, if any, you envisage.

INTRODUCTION

With the progression of global warming it is predicted that the incidence of heatwave will increase. This natural phenomenon produces high temperatures, 24 hours a day, over many days or even weeks. During such prolonged periods of heat, morbidity and mortality attributed to causes such as dehydration, cardiovascular, cerebrovascular and respiratory events increase substantially. Specific adverse health outcomes associated with high environmental temperatures include:

➤ heat stroke
➤ heat exhaustion
➤ heat syncope
➤ heat cramps.[1]

Those at increased risk are:
➤ older people
➤ infants
➤ the frail
➤ the individual with chronic health conditions.

People with mental health disorders, alcohol dependence, drug dependence and those taking prescribed medications such as lithium, neuroleptic and anticholinergic drugs are also at an increased risk.[2-6] This population often experiences poorer overall health, has fewer social supports, and higher rates of mortality and morbidity.[7] Those with a combination of these illnesses, and taking combinations of medications, are at even greater risk.

During periods of extreme temperatures, there is a rapid increase in demand for ambulance and hospital emergency services.[5] As a heatwave continues the capacity of these services to meet such high demand is often seriously compromised. This may result in extended response times, overstretched or even non-existent services.

Adverse health outcomes from heatwaves can be avoided. All professionals (mental health, alcohol treatment, drug treatment, primary health and welfare) have a responsibility to increase the capability and resilience of individuals to manage their health and safety during a heatwave. This discussion raises the importance of the mental health–substance use professional to provide extra assistance, assessments and monitoring when individuals lack the capacity or resources to protect themselves at these times of extreme temperature.

HEATWAVE STUDIES

The majority of these studies have been conducted in South Australia. South Australia is the driest state on the driest inhabited continent (Antarctica is the driest continent).[8] There are two perspectives to consider. The summers are long and the risk of heatwaves in the South Australian region is high. The population is regularly put under stress. Each year there is a high likelihood of many heat-related illnesses. However, it should be considered that the South Australian population have the experience and a continued expectation of heatwaves. Heatwaves can occur in many different regions of the world. People living in cooler climates that unexpectedly experience the occasional heatwave may be less acclimatised with greater negative consequences.

One of the first studies was undertaken in Adelaide, South Australia to ascertain and describe the impact of high environmental temperature on referral loads in a major metropolitan hospital emergency department.[2] The study reported a number of important findings in relation to the types of heat-related presentations for acute medical care and high-risk groups. Multiple medications and concurrent physical illnesses were common in this group. From this study, the authors developed and promoted a standardised emergency treatment response plan for heat stress presentations to emergency departments.[2]

Another study investigated the morbidity and mortality associated with heatwaves in metropolitan Adelaide, South Australia.[5] They analysed ambulance statistics, hospital admissions and mortality data over a 13-year period. The groups identified to be most at risk in heatwave conditions were those with a mental illness across *all* age groups, and those with renal disease in the *older* age groups.

A further study, in Adelaide, examined mental, behavioural and cognitive disorders that may be triggered or exacerbated by heatwaves. Two issues concerning the effects of heat on mental illness were identified.[6]

1   That the nature of the mental disorder could be a risk factor for heat-related morbidity and mortality (*see* Box 14.1). Senility was included in this study because cognitive impairment of the elderly and admissions for senility did increase during heatwave periods.[6]

BOX 14.1 Specific nosologic subgroups for which an increase in admissions was evident[6]

These include:
- organic, including symptomatic mental disorders
- dementia
- mood (affective) disorders
- neurotic, stress-related, somatoform disorders
- disorders of psychological development.

2   That a heatwave may exacerbate pre-existing mental health conditions in general. The authors[6] cite a 2007 study that found having a pre-existing mental illness can more than triple the risk of death during a heatwave and that taking psychotropic medication nearly doubles the risk.[9] However, the study acknowledged the limitations of a small sample size and suggested caution in interpreting the results.[6] For instance, they found that a significant proportion of deaths occurred due to psychoactive substance use in females but not males during this period. Such findings warrant further validation in larger studies. It was suggested that, in general, heat-related illnesses may be under-diagnosed.[6] The study concluded by suggesting that episodes of extreme heat pose a salient risk to the health and safety of the mentally ill.[6]

DISCUSSION

Within the health disaster management literature, heatwaves are described as natural events, which may or may not become disasters. A disaster is when there is serious disruption to the functioning of society, with widespread human, infrastructure, material or environmental losses that exceed the ability of an affected society to cope using its own resources. A natural event considered a disaster in one society may be manageable in the context of another society.[10] While Australia has a long history of heatwaves, and lessons have been learnt, heatwave management particularly for the most vulnerable members of the community can always be improved.

Impact on emergency service delivery

The over-extension of acute healthcare and emergency services is an important issue. During February 2009, Adelaide experienced a heatwave of over a week, which significantly disrupted the functioning of its health and emergency services, electricity supply and transport. The media reported that up to 30 suspected heat-related deaths had occurred during the week of the heatwave.[11]

The growing recognition that major acute healthcare systems may not be able to provide the help required suggests that the community needs to become more independently resourced to withstand the impact of weather extremes, such as heatwaves. It is very important that all professionals take the time to consider and discuss what would be required to assist both themselves and the individual to prepare for extremes in weather conditions related to his/her country's environment. This is because power, transport and emergency service access may be severely affected, leaving people unable to rely on the availability of these services.

Heat effects on the body

To be able to understand the nature of an appropriate healthcare response it is important to have an understanding about how heat affects the body and why people with mental health and substance use conditions are at particular and serious risk from heat-related illness. This next section briefly considers the issue of heat stress and looks at appropriate interventions.

Heat stress

Heat stress is a continuum of physical illnesses relating to the body's inability to cope with exposure to excessive heat. These physical illnesses include:
➤ heat-induced dehydration
➤ rash
➤ cramps
➤ syncope
➤ exhaustion.

They may have many overlapping diagnostic features. The most severe form of heat-related stress is heat stroke and is defined as a body temperature higher than 40.5°C and associated with neurologic dysfunction and absence of sweating.[12,13]

Body temperature is maintained at a constant level by the central nervous system (brain), whereby the hypothalamus functions as a thermostat, guiding the body through the mechanisms of heat production or dissipation. The appropriate physiological response to heat includes dilatation of the peripheral venous system to increase blood flow to the skin. Skin is the major heat dissipating organ and increased blood flow to the skin releases more heat. Another appropriate physiological response is the stimulation of the endocrine sweat glands to produce more sweat.[12–14]

HEAT REGULATION

In more detail, heat is lost and gained from the human body in four ways:
1 conduction
2 convection
3 radiation
4 evaporation.

These mechanisms require a functioning integumentary (skin) system, and autonomic nervous system to provide homeostasis. In addition to these autonomic processes, in order to survive the person may be required to respond to their environment by:
➤ increasing fluid intake (non-alcoholic) to prevent dehydration
➤ removing amounts of clothing
➤ relocating to a cooler or warmer environment.[12]

At high ambient temperatures conduction becomes the least important mechanism for cooling. Evaporation, on the other hand, becomes the most effective mechanism for heat loss. The efficacy of evaporation depends on a number of factors:
➤ condition of the skin and sweat glands

➤ function of the lungs
➤ ambient temperature
➤ humidity
➤ air movement.

The more sweat a person can produce the better the body's ability to dissipate heat through evaporation. The exception to this is when the ambient humidity exceeds 75%.[12] In this situation, if a person's body temperature is elevated, high humidity will prevent the body from dissipating heat through the mechanism of evaporation. This could lead to heat exhaustion or heat stroke, particularly if the person is unable to, or does not change their responses to, counteract their environmental circumstances.

It is important to note that infants have an immature thermoregulatory system. Another group at risk, the elderly, have impaired perception of temperature changes in their bodies, impaired perception of ambient temperatures and a decreased capacity to sweat.[12]

There are a number of circumstances that may prevent the body's natural cooling system from working well. These include:
➤ high environmental temperatures with high humidity
➤ over-dressing
➤ mental or physical inability to respond to and modify the environment (e.g. removing clothes, opening windows, initiating air-conditioning, showering).

Other circumstances include:
➤ changes to the skin through ageing
➤ hypothalamic (hormone) dysfunction
➤ heart, lung or kidney disease
➤ being unable to perspire due to burns or particular medications.[14]

THERMOREGULATORY SIDE-EFFECTS
Psychiatric medications
People with a mental illness are at increased risk of heat-related illnesses.[15] There are three reasons for this.
1 They may have an underlying physical pathology associated with the mental illness, e.g. dysfunction of thermoregulation associated with schizophrenia.[16]
2 They may be more vulnerable due to effects of their prescribed psychiatric medications.
3 The physical or mental impairment associated with their mental illness may affect their ability to recognise, cope and adapt to the change in environmental temperatures.

Neuroleptic (older and newer generations of antipsychotics) and anticholinergic (antiparkinsonian) medications have a well-recognised association with heat intolerance and heat stroke.[15,17] The pathophysiological mechanisms responsible for these syndromes involve serotonin, dopamine and noradrenalin suppressing the function of the thermoregulatory centre in the anterior hypothalamus and causing anhydrosis (loss of perspirative ability to dissipate heat). Interestingly, the suppression of activity in the thermoregulatory centre can produce either hypothermia or hyperthermia, depending on the ambient temperature. These medications also cause cutaneous vasoconstriction and the amount of heat dissipated by convection and radiation wwis reduced.[15,18]

Serotonergic syndrome is a toxin-induced potentially life-threatening adverse drug reaction that results from therapeutic drug use, intentional self-poisoning or inadvertent interactions between drugs.[19] One of its cardinal signs is hyperthermia. The mechanism is complex and involves interaction between the environment, central catecholamine release (noradrenalin, dopamine and serotonin), the hypothalamic-pituitary-thyroid-adrenal axis, the sympathetic nervous system and skeletal muscle.[19–21] Any drug that is capable of increasing the concentration of serotonin in the central nervous system has the potential to cause this syndrome. This includes the older tricyclic antidepressants, the newer generation serotonin specific reuptake inhibitors, serotonin and noradrenalin reuptake inhibitors, and various drugs of dependence.

The excess of serotonin produces a broad spectrum of clinical findings that may range from barely perceptible to lethal, and is exacerbated by heatwave conditions.[19,20]

Lithium is a naturally occurring salt. When administered for the treatment of bipolar disorder, it may interfere with the regulation of sodium and water levels in the body and can cause dehydration readily. Heatwaves may also contribute to the development of dehydration. Therefore, people maintained on lithium during heatwaves are at heightened risk.

Regular serum level tests and the monitoring of thyroid and kidney function for abnormalities are important when maintained on lithium. This is of particular importance during heatwaves. When people are commenced on lithium therapy, they should be advised to remain well hydrated at all times, especially during periods of prolonged hot weather. The individual should be advised to monitor thirst, and drink accordingly to counteract the electrolyte imbalances that might otherwise ensue.

Dehydration can result in increasing lithium levels and lithium toxicity. Toxic effects include:

➤ tremor
➤ ataxia – gross lack of coordination of muscle movements
➤ dysarthria – motor speech disorder characterised by poor articulation
➤ nystagmus – involuntary eye movements causing a degree of vision impairment
➤ renal impairment
➤ convulsions.

If there is evidence of toxicity, the person should cease taking lithium and immediately seek medical advice.

Alcohol and other drugs

Alcohol and opioid use increase cutaneous vasodilation and increase perspiration. This lowers overall body temperature but contributes to dehydration. In addition, alcohol acts as a powerful diuretic leading to excessive fluid loss and dehydration. Alcohol and opioid use can contribute directly to hyperthermia.

Sympathomimetics (amphetamines and amphetamine-like substances, e.g. methamphetamine, cocaine and 3,4-methylenedioxymethamphetamine [MDMA – Ecstasy]), elevate body temperature by two main mechanisms:

1   The release of noradrenalin by these drugs act on the vascular alpha-1 adrenorecep-tors to cause vasoconstriction and decrease blood flow to the cutaneous layer of the skin. This reduces heat loss.
2   Sympathomimetics increase muscular activity through agitation and there is a sub-sequent increase in body heat.[22]

As discussed earlier, thermoregulation in the hypothalamus is controlled by serotonin, dopamine and noradrenalin. Direct and indirect stimulation of the hypothalamus by agents such as 3,4-methylenedioxymethamphetamine (MDMA – Ecstasy), meth-amphetamine and cocaine activate the hypothalamic-pituitary-thyroid-adrenal axis, increasing body heat.[19,23]

Decreasing the use of alcohol and other drugs is recommended during heatwaves. However, if the individuals use alcohol and other drugs in these periods, they should also ensure that fluid intake is increased and strategies are employed to remain in the coolest environment possible.

EDUCATING AND PREPARING THE INDIVIDUAL, FAMILY AND CARERS

All mental health and substance use, emergency, primary health and welfare profes-sionals have a responsibility to educate and support the individual, family and carers to understand and manage the individual's health and safety during times of extreme temperatures. The following discussion provides a list of strategies that should be con-sidered in discussion with the individual, family and carers.

➤ The assessments should describe the individual's capacity to self-manage changes with respect to his/her particular:
  — general health status
  — mental health status
  — living circumstances and environment
  — medication
  — drug and alcohol use
  — social and economic risks from extremes in temperature.

This assessment will inform the strategies for the professional(s) and the individual to use when the environment changes, and the weather becomes extremely hot over a longer period of time.

➤ Those who can contact their treating medical team should have their medications reviewed prior to a predicted heatwave.
➤ The professionals need to implement regular daily monitoring of the individual during periods of extreme heat. Regular close monitoring of the individual's mental and physical health status is necessary during a heatwave to prevent and detect deteriorating health, severe illness and risk of sudden death.
➤ Individuals should be encouraged to seek safe shelter in cool places during this time, taking medication and essential belongings along.

➤ It is also recommended that people keep an accessible and secure store of a few days of any prescribed medications in case of enforced isolation
➤ Changing environmental circumstances may increase the risk of complications in pregnancy or deterioration in chronic medical conditions. These include:
— diabetes
— hypertension
— hepatitis A, B and C
— human immunodeficiency virus (HIV)
— cardiac, renal and liver disease.

The professional needs to prioritise the support mechanisms for the individual with these conditions, and inform the individual and family how best to prevent, detect and manage early signs of complications.

FIRST AID TREATMENT RESPONSE
It is important to put into place a range of practical strategies to decrease the impact on ambulance, hospital and other health services at times of increased demand. Any person found suffering from heat stress (*see* Table 14.1) must be responded to immediately by the following actions.
➤ Placing the individual to rest in a cool place or shade.
➤ Loosening all clothing.
➤ Cooling the body with the most effective method available. This could be by applying ice packs in the areas of the groin and armpits. Other methods are a cool shower, immersing in water, or wrapping in damp sheets. It is important to *avoid making the individual too cool* as he/she may start to shiver, and the body will respond by retaining heat.
➤ Observe the person's vital signs, including their level of consciousness (Glasgow Coma Scale[25]).
➤ Undertake a mental status assessment every 5–10 minutes until stable.
➤ Continue oral rehydration of 2 litres maximum of water and the regular monitoring of fluid intake until the person passes urine.
➤ Follow-up treatment requires ongoing hydration and rest in the coolest place until the ambient heat falls to a level of comfort.[12,13,26]
➤ If symptoms persist beyond one hour, or there is recurrent vomiting or worsening of the individual's mental or physical condition, an ambulance should be called immediately.

TABLE 14.1 Summary of heat-related illnesses and first aid response[24]

Condition	Overview	Signs and symptoms	Management
Heat syncope	Heat syncope is a fainting episode or dizziness that usually occurs with prolonged standing or sudden rising from sitting or lying down. Dehydration is a factor that may contribute to feeling dizzy or fainting.	Fainting	Sit or lie the person down in a cool place. If possible elevate the legs for approximately 30 seconds. Encourage to drink water and/or clear juice slowly.[13,26]
Heat cramps	Heat cramps usually affect people who are carrying out heavy or strenuous activity. Sweating depletes the body's salt and moisture levels. The low salt levels in muscles cause painful cramps. Heat cramps may also be a symptom of heat exhaustion.	Heat cramps may include muscle pain and spasms usually in the abdomen, arms and legs.	Stop all activity. Sit or lie the person down in a cool place. Encourage to drink water or clear juice slowly. Do not return to strenuous activity for a few hours or else it may lead to heat exhaustion. Medical attention should be sought if the person has heart problems or is on a low sodium diet, or cramps do not subside within one hour.[13,26]
Heat exhaustion	Heat exhaustion is a warning that the body is overheating. Early intervention to reduce the heat exhaustion within the community setting will prevent hospitalisation for heat stroke. Heat exhaustion is considered a serious form of heat stress.	• Normal or slight increase in body temperature • Headache • Cool clammy pale skin • Sweating • Dry mouth • Thirst • Fatigue, weakness • Feeling dizzy • Nausea and vomiting may occur • Muscle cramps • Weak and rapid pulse.[12,13,26]	All persons found this way should be placed at rest in a cool place or shade. Loosen clothing. Commence cooling the body with the most effective method available. This could be by applying ice packs in the areas of the groin, armpits or by immersion in cool water, cool shower or wrapping in cold sheets. Avoid making them too cool so they start to shiver as this will cause them to retain heat. Observe vital signs, including a mental status assessment, every 5–10 minutes until stable. Oral rehydration of 2 litres maximum per day of water. Keep monitoring fluids until the person passes urine. Persistent symptoms beyond one hour, recurrent equire an ambulance to be called and attendance at an emergency department. Follow-up requires rest and hydration in the coolest place possible for 24 hours.[12,13,26]

(continued)

Condition	Overview	Signs and symptoms	Management
Heat stroke	Heat stroke is a serious public health problem. With heat stroke, body organs start to overheat. If heat increase continues, the organs will cease functioning. Without treatment death will occur.	Signs and symptoms can occur suddenly with little warning. • Very high body temperature over 41°C • Hot, dry, red skin • No sweating • Throbbing headache • Weak and rapid pulse • Tachypnoea • Hypotension • Confusion, hallucinations, irritability • Convulsions • Ataxia • Slurred speech • Involuntary bowel movement • Loss of consciousness.[12,13,26]	Call an ambulance. All persons found this way should be placed at rest in a cool place or shade. Loosen clothing. Commence cooling the body with the most effective method available. This could be by applying ice packs in the areas of the groin, armpits or by immersion in cool water, cool shower or wrapping in cold sheets until the ambulance arrives or medical assistance is obtained. Observe vital signs, including a mental status assessment, every 5–10 minutes. If possible and there is minimal likelihood of vomiting, commence oral rehydration of 2 litres maximum of water.[12,13,26]
	Exertional heat stroke can occur in people who perform intense prolonged physical activity, particularly in hot weather. Athletes are one of the high-risk groups for exertional heat stroke. They may undertake strenuous physical activity producing high levels of metabolic heat for extended durations, causing their bodies to overheat. They are at increased risk of heat stroke during hot and humid weather.		On arrival at the emergency department intravenous rehydration will commence, and oxygen administered as needed to maintain $SaO_2 > 95\%$. Cooling the body will continue if temperature is over 41°C, with immersion in ice water or soaking the skin in cool or ice-cold sheets and ice packs. Vital signs will continue to be monitored as well as the mental status every 5–10 minutes until stable and body temperature is below 38.5°C. It is important to stop aggressive cooling when the body temperature starts to drop, to avoid hypothermia.
	Non-exertional heat stroke more commonly affects sedentary older people, persons with a chronic illness and very young persons during environmental heatwaves.		Urine samples will be checked for the presence of myoglobinuria. Myoglobin is normally present in the muscle cells as a reserve of oxygen. When present in the urine it is indicative of rhabdomyolysis or muscle destruction. If this occurs consideration must be given for further hospitalisation.[13]
	Importantly, heat stroke is associated with a high morbidity and mortality especially when treatment is delayed.		

Alcohol and drug withdrawal

Another potential complication of extreme weather is unplanned alcohol or drug withdrawal. During a heatwave, individuals may not be able to access their alcohol or other drugs, prescribed pain medication (often opioids) or opioid maintenance therapy (methadone or buprenorphine). Alcohol withdrawal in particular may be life-threatening due to electrolyte and metabolic imbalance. This would be exacerbated by the presence of heat stress. One suggested intervention in such circumstances is an emergency withdrawal kit. This may be appropriate for heatwaves and other natural disasters.[27] Such a kit would include a short supply of symptomatic withdrawal medication such as the following.

1   Paracetamol: for pain and body discomfort.
2   Metoclopramide: for nausea and vomiting.
3   Buscopan (scopolamine butylbromide): an anti-spasmodic that relieves abdominal muscle cramps.
4   Orphenadrine: anticholinergic that relieves leg muscle cramps.
5   Loperamide: opioid that does not cross the blood–brain barrier but relieves diarrhoea.
6   Thiamine: vitamin replacement to prevent Wernicke–Korsakoff syndrome.

Drugs that **should not be included** in the withdrawal kit include the following.
➤ Diazepam: due to its popular appeal as an anxiolytic.
➤ Clonidine: lowers blood pressure. Some people are hypotensive as a result of the medical condition. Heatwaves may cause dehydration which can exacerbate the hypotension. Clonidine may then potentiate the existing hypotension.

CONCLUSION

Heatwaves greatly increase the risk of death and serious illness among those experiencing mental health–substance use problems. The individual who has poor physical health is particularly vulnerable. The risks are exacerbated when extended power blackouts occur and essential services are overstretched. These events impact particularly on:
➤ the homeless
➤ those lacking adequate shelter
➤ sufficient supply of fluids
➤ those relying on public transport. A functioning public transport system may be the essential factor for survival for the individual requiring daily shopping, medical appointments and prescribed medications for mental health or drug dependence conditions.

All professionals (mental health, substance use treatment, primary health and welfare), have a responsibility to discuss these issues with the individual and establish an emergency management plan to keep that person well in preparation for extreme temperatures.

POST-READING EXERCISE 14.1

> **Time: 15 minutes**
> - What is the difference between a disaster and an event?
> - Why are people with mental health and substance use conditions at particular and serious risk during an episode of extreme heat?
> - What other groups are more at risk from heat-related illness and why?
> - What four ways is the body temperature regulated and maintained?
> - What are the three reasons people with a mental illness are at increased risk of heat-related illnesses?
> - What psychiatric medications increase the risk of a heat-related illness and why?
> - What would be your first aid response for heat-related illness?
> - Make a list of what you would discuss with the individual, family and carer to assist them to be prepared for a heatwave.

REFERENCES

1 Landesman L, Veenma T. *Natural Disasters. Disaster nursing and emergency preparedness, for chemical, biological and radiological terrorism and other hazards.* New York, NY: Springer Publishing Company; 2006.

2 Faunt JD, Wilkinson TJ, Aplin P, *et al.* The effete in the heat: heat-related hospital presentations during a ten day heat wave. *Aust N Z J Med.* 1995; **25**: 117–21.

3 Weir E. Heat wave: first, protect the vulnerable. *Can Med Assoc J.* 2002; **167**: 169.

4 Kovats RS, Kristie LE. Heatwaves and public health in Europe. *Eur J Public Health.* 2006; **16**: 592–9.

5 Nitschke M, Tucker GR, Bi P. Morbidity and mortality during heatwaves in metropolitan Adelaide. *Med J Aust.* 2007; **187**: 662–5.

6 Hansen A, Bi P, Nitschke M, *et al.* The effect of heat waves on mental health in a temperate Australian city. *Environ Health Perspect.* 2008; **116**: 1369–75. p. 1372.

7 Australian Bureau of Statistics. *Measures of Australia's Progress: summary indicators, 2009.* Available at: www.abs.gov.au/AUSSTATS/abs@.nsf/Lookup/1383.0.55.001Main+Features102009 (accessed 22 February 2010).

8 Australian Bureau of Meteorology. *Australian Climate Extremes – time series graphs, 2009.* Available at: www.bom.gov.au/cgi-bin/climate/change/extremes/timeseries.cgi (accessed 22 February 2010).

9 Bouchama A, Dehbi M, Mohamed G, *et al.* Prognostic factors in heat wave-related deaths. *Arch Int Med.* 2007; **167**: 2170–6.

10 Sundnes KO. Health disaster management: guidelines for evaluation and research in the Utstein style: executive summary. Task Force on Quality Control of Disaster Management. *Prehosp Disaster Med.* 1999; **14**: 43–52.

11 Crouch B, Kyriacou K, Owen M. Sudden deaths rise across Adelaide amid 40C-plus heatwave. *Adelaide Now.* 31 Jan; 2009.

12 Helman R, Habal R. Heatstroke. *eMedicine Emergency Medicine.* November 2007. Available at: www.medscape.com/emergencymedicine (accessed 12 March 2010).

13 Carter III R, Cheuvront S, Sawka M. *Heat Related Illnesses.* Sports Science Library; 2008. Available at: www.gssiweb.com/Article_Detail.aspx?articleid=728 (accessed 22 February 2010).

14 Cree L, Rischmiller S. *Science in Nursing,* Melbourne, VIC: Holt-Saunders Pty Ltd; 1986.

15 Reilly TH, Kirk MA. Atypical antipsychotics and newer antidepressants. *Emerg Med Clin North Am.* 2007; **25**: 477–97.

16 Hermesh H, Shiloh R, Epstein Y, *et al.* Heat intolerance in patients with chronic schizophrenia maintained with antipsychotic drugs. *Am J Psychiatry.* 2000; **157**: 1327–9.

17 Bhanushali MJ, Tuite PJ. The evaluation and management of patients with neuroleptic malignant syndrome. *Neurol Clin.* 2004; **22**: 389–411.

18 Stadnyk AN, Glezos JD. Drug-induced heat stroke. *Can Med Assoc J.* 1983; **128**: 957–9.

19 Eyer F, Zilker T. Bench-to-bedside review: mechanisms and management of hyperthermia due to toxicity. *Crit Care.* 2007; **11**: 236.

20 Boyer EW, Shannon M. The serotonin syndrome. *N Engl J Med.* 2005; **352**: 1112–20.

21 Rusyniak DE, Sprague JE. Hyperthermic syndromes induced by toxins. *Clin Lab Med.* 2006; **26**(1): 165–84.

22 Martinez M, Devenport L, Saussy J, *et al.* Drug-associated heat stroke. *South Med J.* 2002; **95**: 799–802.

23 Fernandez F, Aguerre S, Mormede P, *et al.* Influences of the corticotropic axis and sympathetic activity on neurochemical consequences of 3,4-methylenedioxymethamphetamine (MDMA) administration in Fischer 344 rats. *Eur J Neurosci.* 2002; **16**(4): 607–18.

24 Mateer J, Cusack J, Ranse J. Environmental emergencies and pandemics. In: Curtis K, Ramsden C. *Emergency and Trauma Care.* Chatswood, NSW: Elsevier (Australia); in press.

25 National Institute for Health and Clinical Excellence. *Head Injury: observation and proformas and Glasgow Coma Scale.* Available at: http://guidance.nice.org.uk/index.jsp?action =download&o=36266 (accessed 22 February 2010).

26 National Institute for Occupational Safety and Health. *Heat Stress.* 2009. Available at: www.cdc. gov/niosh/topics/heatstress (accessed 22 February 2010).

27 Neild R. *Emergency Withdrawal Kit.* Personal communication; 2009.

TO LEARN MORE

Alcohol, Tobacco and Other Drugs Guidelines for Nurses and Midwives: Clinical Guidelines are available for download at: www.dassa.sa.gov.au/site/page.cfm?u=230

Guidelines on the management of co-occurring alcohol and other drug and mental health conditions in alcohol and other drug treatment settings are available for download at: http://ndarc.med. unsw.edu.au/NDARCWeb.nsf/page/Comorbidity+Guidelines

Useful chapters

The *Mental Health–Substance Use* series comprises six books. To develop knowledge and understanding chapters are interlinked, building and exploring specific areas. It is hoped the following will help readers locate relevant chapters easily.

BOOK 2: DEVELOPING SERVICES IN MENTAL HEALTH–SUBSTANCE USE

BOOK 3: RESPONDING IN MENTAL HEALTH–SUBSTANCE USE

BOOK 6: PRACTICE IN MENTAL HEALTH–SUBSTANCE USE

Useful contacts

Collated by Jo Cooper

- Addiction Arena – www.addictionarena.com
- Addiction Medicine – http://listserv.icors.org/SCRIPTS/WA-ICORS.EXE?A0=ADD_MED
- Addiction Rehabilitation Facilities – www.arf.org/isd/bib/mental.html
- Addiction Technology Transfer Center – www.nattc.org/index.html
- Addiction Today – www.addictiontoday.org
- Alcohol and Alcohol Problems Science Database – http://etoh.niaaa.nih.gov
- Alcohol and Drug History Society – http://historyofalcoholanddrugs.typepad.com
- Alcohol Concern – www.alcoholconcern.org.uk/servlets/home
- Alcohol Drugs and Development – www.add-resources.org
- Alcohol Focus Scotland – www.alcohol-focus-scotland.org.uk
- Alcohol Misuse (Department of Health) – www.dh.gov.uk/en/Publichealth/Healthimprovement/Alcoholmisuse/index.htm
- Alcohol Reports – www.alcoholreports.blogspot.com
- Alcohol, Other Drugs and Health: Current Evidence – www.bu.edu/aodhealth/index.html
- Alcoholics Anonymous – www.aa.org
- Alcoholism and Substance Abuse Providers – www.asapnys.org
- American Psychiatric Association – www.psych.org
- American Society of Addiction Medicine – www.asam.org/CMEonline.html
- ATTC Network – www.attcnetwork.org/index.asp
- Australasian Professional Society on Alcohol and other Drugs – www.apsad.org.au
- Australian Drug Foundation – www.adf.org.au
- Australian Drug Information Network – www.adin.com.au/content.asp?Document_ID=1
- Australian Government Department of Health and Ageing:
    - Alcohol – www.alcohol.gov.au
    - Illicit drugs – www.health.gov.au/internet/main/publishing.nsf/Content/health-pubhlth-strateg-drugs-illicit-index.htm
    - Mental health – www.health.gov.au/internet/main/Publishing.nsf/Content/mental-pubs-n-pol08
- Australian Professional Society on Alcohol and Other Drugs – www.apsad2008.com
- Berman Institute of Bioethics – www.bioethicsinstitute.org
- Best Practice Portal – www.emcdda.europa.eu/best-practice
- BioMed Central – www.biomedcentral.com
- Brain Injury Australia – www.bia.net.au
- Brain Trauma Foundation – www.braintrauma.org
- Brief Addiction Science Information Source – www.basisonline.org/2007/10/toward-a-balanc.html

- Campaign for Effective Prevention and Treatment of Addiction – www.solutionstodrugs.com/index.htm
- CEBMH www.cebmh.com
- Centre for Addiction and Mental Health Services – www.camh.net
- Centre for Clinical and Academic Workforce Innovation: Tel: 01623 819140: email: ccawi@lincoln.ac.uk
- Centre for HIV & Sexual Health, Sheffield Primary Care NHS Trust – www.sexualhealthsheffield.nhs.uk
- Centre for Independent Thought – www.centerforindependentthought.org
- Centre for Mental Health – www.scmh.org.uk/index.aspx
- Clan Unity – www.clan-unity.co.uk
- Committee on Publication Ethics – http://publicationethics.org
- Communities of Practice for Local Government – www.communities.idea.gov.uk
- Community Based Care Nurses Association – www.communitynursingnetwork.org/
- Comorbid Mental Health and Substance Misuse in Scotland – www.drugmisuse.isdscotland.org/smrt/smrt.htm: www.scotland.gov.uk/Resource /Doc/127665/0030583.pdf
- Co-occurring mental and substance abuse disorders: a guide for mental health planning and advisory councils – http://download.ncadi.samhsa.gov/ken/pdf/NMH03-0146/NMH03-0146.pdf
- Creative Commons – http://creativecommons.org
- Daily Dose: Drug and Alcohol News from Around the World – http://dailydose.net
- Dartmouth Psychiatric Research Centre – dms.dartmouth.edu/prc/dual
- Department of Health – www.dh.gov.uk
- Department of Primary Health Care – www.primarycare.ox.ac.uk/research/dipex
- Doctors.net.uk – www.doctors.org.uk
- Drink and Drugs News – www.drinkanddrugs.net
- Drinks Media Wire – www.drinksmediawire.com/afficher_cdp.asp?id=2625&lng=2
- Drug and Alcohol Findings – http://findings.org.uk
- Drug and Alcohol Nurses Australia – www.danaonline.org
- Drug and Alcohol Services, South Australia – www.dassa.sa.gov.au
- Drug Misuse Information Scotland – www.drugmisuse.isdscotland.org/news/events.htm
- DrugInfo Clearing House – http://druginfo.adf.org.au
- Drugs and Mental Health –www.thesite.org/drinkanddrugs/drugsafety/drugsandyourbody/drugsandmentalhealth
- Drugtext Internet Library – www.drugtext.org
- Dual Diagnosis – Australia and New Zealand – www.dualdiagnosis.org.au/home
- Dual Diagnosis – www.hoseahouse.org/infirmary/dualdx.html
- Dual Diagnosis Support Victoria – http://dualdiagnosis.ning.com
- Dual Diagnosis Toolkit – www.rethink.org/dualdiagnosis/toolkit.html
- Dual Diagnosis Website – http://users.erols.com/ksciacca
- Enter Mental Health: www.entermentalhealth.net/home2.html
- European Alcohol Policy Alliance – www.eurocare.org
- European Association for the Treatment of Addiction – www.eata.org.uk
- European Federation of Nurses Associations – www.efnweb.org/version1/en/index.html
- European Monitoring Centre for Drugs and Drug Addiction – www.emcdda.europa.eu
- European Working Group on Drugs Oriented Research – www.dass.stir.ac.uk/old-site/sections/scot-ad/ewodor.htm
- Eye Movement Desensitisation and Reprocessing Training Workshops – www.emdrworkshops.com
- Faces and Voices of Recovery – www.facesandvoicesofrecovery.org

- Federation of Drug and Alcohol Professionals – www.fdap.org.uk/certification/dap.html
- Global Alcohol Harm Reduction Network – http://groups.google.com/group/gahr-net?hl=en&pli=1
- Global Health Council – www.globalhealth.org
- Guardian UK provides a website 'The most useful websites on dual diagnosis' – http://society.guardian.co.uk/mentalhealth/page/0,8149,688817,00.html
- Headway – www.headway.org.uk
- Health and Safety Executive (HSE) – www.hse.gov.uk/stress
- HIT – www.hit.org.uk
- Horatio – European Psychiatric Nurses – www.horatio-web.eu
- Hub of Commissioned Alcohol Projects and Policies – www.hubcapp.org.uk
- Inexcess, in search of recovery – www.inexcess.tv
- International Brain Injury Association – www.internationalbrain.org
- International Centre for Alcohol Policies – www.icap.org
- International Council of Nurses – www.icn.ch
- International Council on Alcohol and Addictions – www.icaa.ch
- International Drug Policy Consortium – www.idpc.net
- International Harm Reduction Association – www.ihra.net
- International Nurses Society on Addictions – www.intnsa.org
- International Society of Addiction Journal Editors – www.parint.org/isajewebsite/index.htm
- IVO, scientific institute in lifestyle, addiction and social developments – www.ivo.nl
- James Lind Library – www.jameslindlibrary.org
- Join Together (Advancing Effective Alcohol and Drug Policy, Prevention and Treatment) – www.jointogether.org
- Links to Other Websites Related to Addiction – www.well.com/user/woa/aodsites.htm
- Madness and Literature Network – www.madnessandliterature.org/index.php
- Medical Council on Alcohol – www.m-c-a.org.uk
- Medline Plus – www.nlm.nih.gov/medlineplus/dualdiagnosis.html
- Mental Health (About.com) – http://mentalhealth.about.com
- Mental Health and Addiction (Centre for Addiction and Mental Health) – www.camh.net/MHA101
- Mental Health and Addictions Research Network – www.mhanet.ca/index.php
- Mental Health Europe – www.mhe-sme.org/en.html
- Mental Health Information for All (RCPSYCH) – www.rcpsych.ac.uk/mentalhealthinfoforall.aspx
- Mental Health Forum – www.mentalhealthforum.net/forum
- Mental Health Foundation – www.mentalhealth.org.uk/welcome
- Mental Health in Higher Education – www.mhhe.heacademy.ac.uk/sitepages/educators/?edid=239
- Mental Health Policy Implementation Guide: dual diagnosis good practice guide – www.dh.gov.uk/en/Publicationsandstatistics/Publications/PublicationsPolicyAndGuidance/DH_4009058
- Mental Health Research Network – http://homepages.ed.ac.uk/mhrn
- Middlesex University Dual Diagnosis Courses – www.mdx.ac.uk/courses/postgraduate/nursing_midwifery_health/index/aspx
- MIND – www.mind.org.uk
- Ministry of Justice (National Offender Management Service) – www.justice.gov.uk/about/noms.htm
- Mood Disorders Association of Canada – www.mooddisorderscanada.ca
- Motivational Interventions for Drugs and Alcohol Misuse in Schizophrenia – www.midastrial.ac.uk

- Motivational Interviewing – www.motivationalinterview.org
- National Alliance on Mental Illness (US) – www.nami.org
- National Centre for Education and Training on Addiction Australia – www.nceta.flinders.edu.au/index.html
- National Comorbidity Initiative Australia – www.health.gov.au/internet/main/publishing.nsf/Content/health-pubhlth-publicat-document-metadata-comorbidity.htm
- National Consortium of Consultant Nurses in Dual Diagnosis and Substance Use – www.dualdiagnosis.co.uk
- National Drug & Alcohol Research Centre – http://ndarc.med.unsw.edu.au/NDARCWeb.nsf
- National Drug Research Institute – http://ndri.curtin.edu.au
- National Health Service – www.justice.gov.uk/about/noms.htm
- National Health Service Litigation Authority – www.nhsla.com/home.htm
- National Institute for Health and Clinical Excellence – www.nice.org.uk
- National Institute of Mental Health – www.nimh.nih.gov
- National Institute on Alcohol Abuse and Alcoholism – www.niaaa.nih.gov
- National Institute on Drug Abuse – www.drugabuse.gov/nidahome.html
- National Treatment Agency for Substance Misuse – www.nta.nhs.uk
- New Directions in the Study of Alcohol – www.newdirections.org.uk
- New South Wales Health Dual Disorders resources – www.druginfo.nsw.gov.au/illicit_drugs
- NHS CHOICES – www.nhs.uk/conditions/heat-exhaustion-and-heatstroke/Pages/Introduction.aspx
- NHS Institute for Innovation and Improvement – www.institute.nhs.uk
- Nordic Council on Dual Diagnosis – www.norden.org/en/areas-of-co-operation/alcohol-and-drugs
- O'Grady CP, Skinner WJ. *Family Guide to Concurrent Disorders* – www.camh.net/Publications/Resources for Professionals/Partnering with families/partnering families famguide.pdf
- Partnership in Coping – www.pinc-recovery.com
- PROGRESS – National Consortium of Consultant Nurses in Dual Diagnosis and Substance Use – www.dualdiagnosis.co.uk
- Promoting Adult Learning – www.niace.org.uk/current-work/area/mental-health
- Psychiatric Nursing – www.citypsych.com/index.html
- Psychminded – www.psychminded.co.uk
- Public Access (National Institutes of Health) – http://publicaccess.nih.gov/index.htm
- Rethink (UK) – www.rethink.org/dualdiagnosis
- Royal College of General Practitioners – www.rcgp.org.uk
- Royal College of Psychiatrists – www.rcpsych.ac.uk
- Royal Society for the Encouragement of Arts – www.thersa.org/home
- SANE Australia – www.sane.org
- Schizophrenia Society of Canada – www.schizophrenia.ca
- Scholarship Society – www.scholarshipsociety.org
- Scottish Addiction Studies – www.dass.stir.ac.uk/sections/showsection.php?id=4
- Scottish Addiction Studies Library – www.drugslibrary.stir.ac.uk
- Social Care Institute for Excellence – www.scie.org.uk
- Social Care Online – www.scie-socialcareonline.org.uk
- Society for the Study of Addiction – www.addiction-ssa.org
- Spanish Peaks Mental Health Centre – www.spmhc.org
- Stigma in Mental Health and Addiction – www.cmhanl.ca/pdf/Stigma.pdf
- Substance Abuse and Mental Health Center toolkit for integrated treatment for co-occurring disorders – http://mentalhealth.samhsa.gov/cmhs/CommunitySupport/toolkits/cooccurring
- Substance Abuse and Mental Health Data Archive – www.icpsr.umich.edu/SAMHDA

- Substance Abuse and Mental Health Services Administration – www.samhsa.gov
- Substance Misuse Management in General Practice – www.smmgp.org.uk
- The Addiction Project – www.theaddictionproject.com
- The Clifford Beers Foundation (promoting mental health) – www.cliffordbeersfoundation.co.uk/jcont91.htm
- The Co-occurring Centre for Excellence (US) – www.coce.samhsa.gov
- The International Community for Hearing Voices – www.intervoiceonline.org
- The International Network of Nurses – www.tinnurses.org
- The International Society for the Study of Drug Policy – www.issdp.org
- The James Lind Alliance Guidebook – www.jlaguidebook.org
- The Management Standards Consultancy – www.themsc.org
- The Mentor Foundation – www.mentorfoundation.org/about_mentor.php?nav=3-27-34-150
- The Methadone Alliance Forum – www.m-alliance.org.uk/forum.html
- The National Centre on Addiction and Substance Abuse – www.casacolumbia.org/templates/Home.aspx?articleid=287&zoneid=32
- The National Drug and Alcohol Research Centre – http://ndarc.med.unsw.edu.au
- The National Institute on Drug Abuse – www.drugabuse.gov/nidahome.htm-l
- The National Treatment Agency – www.nta.nhs.uk
- The Oxford Centre for Neuroethics – www.neuroethics.ox.ac.uk
- The Recovery Workshop – www.recoveryworkshop.com
- The Royal College of Psychiatrists. *Changing Minds Campaign* – www.rcpsych.ac.uk/campaigns/previouscampaigns/changingminds.aspx
- The Sacred Space Foundation – www.sacredspace.org.uk
- The Tidal Model – www.tidal-model.com
- The United Nations Office on Drugs and Crime – www.unodc.org
- The University of Toronto Joint Centre for Bioethics Centre for Addiction and Mental Health Bioethics Service – www.jointcentreforbioethics.ca/partners/camh.shtml
- Tilburg University, Department of Tranzo – www.uvt.nl/tranzo
- Toc H – www.toch-uk.org.uk
- Treatment Improvement Exchange – www.treatment.org
- Trimbos-Institute – centre of expertise on mental health and addiction – www.trimbos.org
- Turning Point – www.turning-point.co.uk
- Tx Director – www.txdirector.com
- UK Database of Uncertainties about the Effects of Treatment – www.library.nhs.uk/DUETs/Default.aspx
- UK Drug Policy Commission – www.ukdpc.org.uk/index.shtml
- UNGASS – www.ungassondrugs.org
- Victorian Alcohol and Drug Association – www.vaada.org.au
- Welcome – Progress – National Consortium of Consultant Nurses in Dual Diagnosis and Substance Use – www.dualdiagnosis.co.uk/Default.ink
- Wired In – Empowering People – http://wiredin.org.uk
- World Health Organization (management of substance abuse) – www.who.int/substance abuse/en
- World Health Organization (Mental Health Policy) – www.who.int/mental_health/policy/en
- World Health Organization: Global Change and Health – www.euro.who.int/globalchange/Topics/20080513_1
- World Medical Association – www.wma.net/en/10home/index.html
- Youth Drug Support, Australia – www.yds.org.au

Index